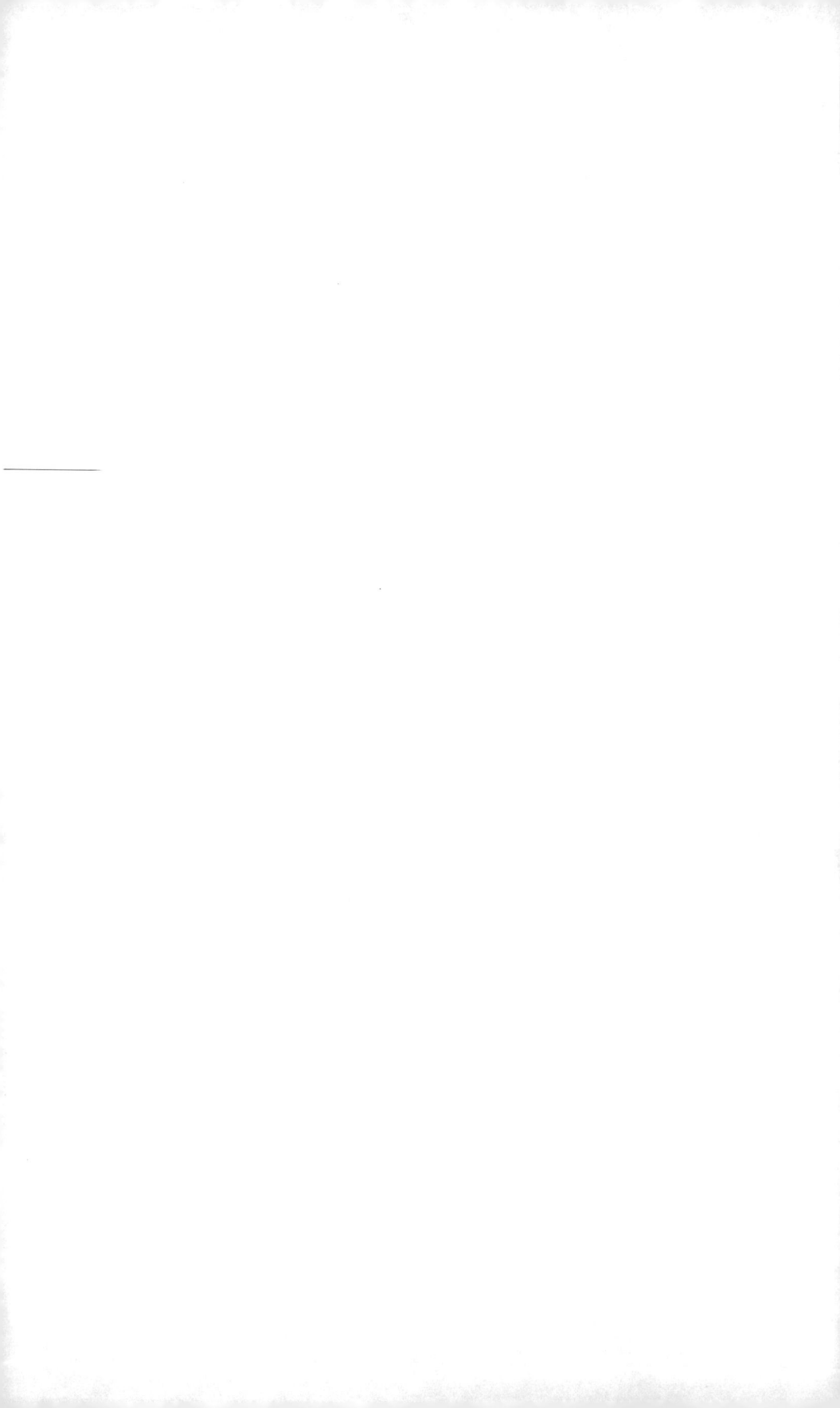

The
Carb
Reset

The Carb Reset

STORE LESS FAT, BURN THE REST,
AND HARNESS THE POWER OF CARBS
TO LOSE WEIGHT

Harley Pasternak, MSc

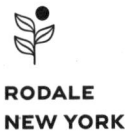

RODALE
NEW YORK

No book can replace the diagnostic expertise and medical advice of a trusted physician. Please be certain to consult with your doctor before making any decisions that affect your health, particularly if you suffer from any medical condition or have any symptoms that may require treatment.

Rodale Books
An imprint of Random House
A division of Penguin Random House LLC
1745 Broadway, New York, NY 10019
rodalebooks.com | randomhousebooks.com
penguinrandomhouse.com

LIBRARY OF CONGRESS CATALOGING-IN-PUBLICATION DATA

ISBN 978-0-593-57881-0
Ebook ISBN 978-0-593-57882-7

Printed in the United States of America on acid-free paper

1st Printing

First Edition

BOOK TEAM: Production editor: Andy Lefkowitz • Managing editor: Allison Fox • Production manager: Richard Elman • Copy editor: Deborah Weiss Geline • Proofreaders: Pam Feinstein, Taylor McGowan, Lori Newhouse, Robin Slutzky, and Marinda Valenti • Indexer: Beverlee Day

Illustrations by Peter Arkle
Freehand Circles art by svetolk/Adobe Stock

The authorized representative in the EU for product safety and compliance is Penguin Random House Ireland, Morrison Chambers, 32 Nassau Street, Dublin D02 YH68, Ireland. https://eu-contact.penguin.ie

For Mila, Bo, Liv, Jess

For all the people who still believe in
evidence-based knowledge, logic, and reality . . .
and still enjoy eating good food

Thank you to Sheila, Marnie, Susie, and Andy

Contents

Introduction

I recently went to an In-N-Out Burger with a friend, and he ordered a double cheeseburger with bacon with extra bacon and mayo and wrapped in lettuce—no bun. Also, no tomato, no ketchup, no red pepper. This was an Atkins-, keto-, and zero-carb-friendly "meal" that had three days'(!) worth of the daily recommendation for saturated fat. When my friend saw the look of horror on my face, he told me to relax; he was eating "animal style" and had lost five pounds in a week. But I knew that it was only a matter of time before he would not be able to sustain the diet and would likely gain back what he lost . . . and more.

For decades, nutrition advice has been stuck in an endless pattern of identifying a problem, taking an extreme stance, and creating a "solution" that ultimately creates more problems than it solves. The pattern is so pervasive that you probably haven't noticed when it's happening, but when we look back, the pattern is as clear as day. One of the consistent aspects of these diets is vilifying one food in favor of another. Different diet; different demon food.

Back in the 1980s and early '90s, it was determined that fat was the problem. Food manufacturers rushed to create "fat-free" products and we—unsuspecting consumers—got peace of mind by reaching for anything that had that label slapped onto it. In my house this meant that breakfast was usually raisin bran cereal (which was marketed at the time as "fat free") with nonfat (skim) milk. Lunch was often a "reduced-fat" turkey sandwich on whole wheat bread with fat-free cheese, mustard, and some pickles with a Fruit Roll-Ups for "dessert." Our dinner repertoire featured a heaping plate of spaghetti and tomato sauce, a stuffed baked potato, or a chicken stir-fry with teriyaki sauce. After dinner we'd treat ourselves to fat-free cookies, licorice, or sorbet. We were deathly afraid of fat and were convinced that if we *ate* fat, we would *be* fat. Carbs, and to a lesser extent proteins, were "safe" foods. They would give us energy, and our waistlines would be kept in check.

Then, in the late 1990s and early 2000s, the United States government's nutritional guidelines determined that fats were no longer the enemy; we were told, instead, that it was potatoes, pasta, rice, bread, many fruits, and some vegetables that were making us fat and unhealthy. Because carbohydrates were the new dietary evil, diets like Atkins that promoted eating fats exploded. More recently, diets like paleo and carnivore picked up the baton from Atkins and continued to fan the flames of our fear of carbs. Even the scientific-sounding ketogenic diet tells us that carbs are to be avoided at all costs. This was the advice that my friend at In-N-Out took to heart.

But why is it that as we have trended away from carbs and sugar, obesity rates have consistently trended upward? It's because deprivation is not sustainable, nor is it particularly healthy. And as you'll find in the pages to come, it is actually the obsessive approach to keeping carbs off our plates that has had the most negatively profound effect. It's time to stop the madness!

A DIET THAT FINALLY WORKS FOR YOU

I know what you're thinking: *"Why is this plan any different from the diets I've criticized above? How can I promise that this is the one that will help you with your weight struggles for good and that you'll finally be able to follow for the long term?"* The answer is simple: with *The Carb Reset* you won't have to give up whole food groups or twist yourself into knots to count calories, fast, or time your meals. You won't have to eliminate anything.

When I talk about a reset, I'm referring to a fresh start with a new perspective. I'm focused on putting you in charge of your health and not feeling controlled by food. This doesn't mean restricting or eliminating entire categories of foods, but it does mean eating foods that help your body work *for* you. For example, protein and fiber and fat give your brain a helpful stop sign. They slow down digestion, help control your blood sugar, make you fuller for longer, and support a healthier metabolism. There are lots of good sources of protein, and you'll learn about those in the following pages, but you'll also discover that precious fiber often hides in carbohydrates—the ones you've probably been studiously avoiding. As *The Carb Reset* suggests right there in the title, it's time to refresh your attitude toward those ingredients.

You'll also need to reset your relationship with high-fat and high-sugar foods. They trigger reward circuits in your brain, cueing you to immediately want more. But they don't fill you up, so you end up eating more than you normally would. However, by resetting what you eat to focus on the right fats, healthy carbs, and limited sugar, you don't run into these issues.

In addition to not restricting whole food groups, *The Carb Reset* embraces *flexibility*. Not restriction. Not sacrifice. Not being miserable without being able to eat your favorite indulgence. Flexibility!

Case in point: I have a not-so-secret daily habit that catches people off guard and often elicits some double takes. Wherever I am, I love going to a great coffee shop and ordering a chocolate chip cookie. I then sit down and take my time enjoying every bite. It's funny to see people who recognize me because they always freak out when I start to eat the cookie. They see the guy who is a nutritionist and personal trainer and who has written several successful weight-loss books knocking back some sugary carbs, and they feel as if they've caught me cheating. They don't realize that I have nothing to hide. If they looked at the rest of my day and saw how my meals are balanced—with carbs, protein, fats, and vegetables—the cookie fits in perfectly fine. Plus, because I hit my steps goal every day and do resistance training regularly, the cookie is merely a drop in the caloric bucket. I eat a chocolate chip cookie almost every day, and I plan on sticking with that habit for the rest of my life.

That cookie is symbolic of how I approach diet and weight loss. If you can't have flexibility in what you eat and eat what you love, there is no pathway to achieving healthy weight loss. The ability to have a cookie (or treat of your choice), along with maintaining balance in your daily meals, is what this book is all about. I'm going to teach you to follow a different path to health from what you may have tried before. The flexibility that allows me to have my favorite chocolate chip cookie is what I want you to bring to your diet and nutrition goals.

> If you can't have flexibility in what you eat and eat what you love, there is no pathway to achieving healthy weight loss.

I've dedicated my life to nutritional science and exercise physiology and have multiple degrees in both. I've been in private practice for thirty-three years, working with some of the most famous people in the world, from massive pop stars like Lady Gaga, Rihanna, Katy Perry, Ariana Grande, Alicia Keys, Adam Levine, and Bono to Hollywood actors including Megan Fox, Robert Downey, Jr., Gwyneth Paltrow, Halle Berry, Kim Kardashian, and many more. Prior to that, I spent nearly a decade at university doing undergraduate and graduate nutritional science and exercise physiology, followed by three years as a nutrition scientist for the military. I've written bestselling nutrition and fitness books and am currently an adjunct professor at the University of Toronto. In other words, I've dedicated my life to helping people lose weight and live longer.

In thirty-plus years, I have seen absolutely every single fad diet come and go—Zone Diet, Pritikin, Atkins, paleo, cabbage soup diet, caveman diet, keto, intermittent fasting, grapefruit diet, Master Cleanse, blood type diet, and dozens more. I've also seen the unfortunate and negative experiences people have had from following these diets—from digestive and sleep issues to severe low blood sugar to initially losing weight and then gaining it back. Unfortunately, people tend to have short memories and forget the negatives they experienced from one fad diet and eagerly move on to another, hoping that this time it will be different and they will lose weight once and for all. But when they run from one diet to the next, each time they end up craving the foods they are told to avoid. Would you rather dream about dessert for the rest of your life or enjoy a chocolate chip cookie? Do you want to fill your plate with spiralized vegetable "noodles" or enjoy a serving of pasta? Would you be surprised to know that you can eat bread *and* have a healthy lean body?

You've been taught to fear foods—including nutrient-dense foods like fruits, vegetables, and grains. It's beautiful and empowering when you realize that food should not be a source of stress and anxiety (both of which make it easier to store fat by influencing hormones and causing chemical changes in your body that make you more likely to overeat).

This diet is truly different. It's a diet that will lead you to the health goals you have been working toward. I like to think of it as the last diet you'll ever need.

HOW TO USE THIS BOOK

In these pages I show you how to easily avoid the most common missteps in dieting and changing eating patterns and to understand exactly what stands between you and the body you desire. Part I helps dispel the myths that have been leading us all in the wrong direction concerning weight loss and health. Chief among these myths is that carbohydrates are bad for you and should not have a place in your diet. That's why this book is called *The Carb Reset*! You've got to reset your understanding of this major macronutrient and make space for it on your plate. I give you background on the science that tells us why the combination of carbs, protein, fats, and vegetables provides the nutrition you need to be healthy, and how the right balance of these foods can help you lose weight.

One of the fundamental pieces of this new approach is to teach you how you can not only burn more fat but store less fat—which will dial down the numbers on the scale and help you look better, feel better, and be in better health. Almost every food has a role in this goal—even sugar—but *especially* carbs, which is yet again a reason for the emphasis on carbs in the title. It's time for you to see how many of the foods you've been missing in the name of losing weight are actually the key to being healthier.

In Part I you also learn how to use my unique approach to selecting balanced portions of essential nutrients for your meals. You can do this by following *The Carb Reset* PATH, a simple way to think about eating without having to stress about calories, weighing your foods, or wondering if you're getting enough of what you need to support your body's needs. **PATH** stands for: a **P**alm of carbohydrates, **A**ll the vegetables, a **T**humb of fat, and a **H**and of protein. I offer guidance on the types of carbs, veggies, fats, and proteins that should find their way onto your plate. You will be happy to know that there is a range to choose from, so you can have a diet that is not only flexible but flavorful. You also gain insight into what may have gotten in the way of your previous attempts at changing the way you eat and receive the tools to overcome the most common roadblocks in your quest for health.

Part II gives you all you need to know to get the right food on your plate with meal plans and recipes to help you eat from all the food groups and enjoy your meals as you reach your health goals.

PREPARE TO SUCCEED!

This plan is different because you will be doing a lot less restricting and a lot more adjusting. Using PATH helps you to set portion sizes in a new way and allows you to fill your plate with a variety of foods, including carbohydrates, and change them up for each meal. Adjusting your diet, and the foods you put on your plate, clears the road to success because you are making choices that work for you. That flexibility—a total reset from the usual deprivation diet—will support and sustain the new way you are eating, and you will be successful in attaining your health and weight-loss goals. These guidelines bring to life the adaptability I use to succeed with my clients, all of whom have different body types and needs.

You can personalize the plan to your preferences, whether that's the foods you enjoy or how many meals you will eat throughout the day. You'll be eating bread, enjoying pasta, and having rice, which will help your body get lean and stay lean. You'll eat protein (your choice of animal- or plant-based). I also encourage you to eat plenty of fruits and vegetables and have included recipes that will help even the most vegetable-resistant person find ways to enjoy plenty of veggies. If you don't want to eat a particular food because you don't enjoy it, then you don't have to.

When people first try this style of eating, they worry that they won't lose weight. They are conditioned to think that severe sacrifices go hand in hand with a diet, and they wonder if *The Carb Reset* has them giving up enough to gain what they want. You may find yourself thinking along these same lines, but I don't want you to worry about being in starvation mode, worry that having too much protein may cause kidney damage, or think that you need to wear a continuous glucose monitor (CGM) to track your blood sugar response to everything you eat. I want you to be free from all of that so you can focus on making a new habit of easy, accessible, sustainable eating principles that you can repeat each day.

I know this approach works—I have thousands of happy clients to show for it—and I've seen that it is a plan that can be followed for life. *The Carb Reset* has been created to address the fact that if a diet is not sustainable and doesn't bring you joy, you are being set up for failure. It is backed by science and my years of experience, and teaches you how to bring balance to the foods you eat, the diet you follow, and your ability to reach your health goals.

Almost everything you've been told about diets so far has taken you farther from the finish line you've been trying to cross. I will get you across the line. Let's get started!

PART I

Getting on the Road to Better, Long-Lasting Health

CHAPTER 1

The Truth About Losing Weight

"*Where did I go wrong?*"

I've been asked this question about weight loss thousands of times. The answer is simple, but it's not what most people think. Diets have taught us to look for a single cause that simultaneously makes losing weight easier and gaining weight harder.

However, the issues of weight gain and loss can't be linked to a single source. To better understand why you gain weight and how you can more effectively lose weight—and keep it off—you need to understand what drives us to eat more (and how to get back in control), why losing weight can feel impossible (when it's not), and how to stop falling for the hype and misinformation of diet trends (and learn what really works).

Here's the truth: *the more restrictive the approach, the more damaging it is to your health*. Need proof? Over the last several decades, more "fringe" diets have emerged than at any time previously—no gluten, no dairy, no grains, no sugar, no carbs, only nighttime eating, no morning eating, and so on. Back in the 1960s and '70s, obesity affected approximately 13 percent of people in the United States. As I write this today, the obesity rate is more than *40 percent!*[1] To state the obvious, these diets don't seem to have had a positive impact.

When people talk about the "best" diet or the best way to lose weight, an important piece of the discussion is often left out—what has been driving our eating behaviors and why that has been pushing us to eat more and gain weight. Global weight gain—which is estimated to cost the world more than $4.3 *trillion* in healthcare costs over the next decade[2]—is the by-product of a food industry that made a subtle, but significant, change about forty years ago. Ever since then, we've been repeating the same mistakes, falling for the same lies, and being manipulated by health food messaging that has made us less healthy.

You are being sold foods that you *think* are healthy and good for you. And when those foods don't make you healthier, you feel like you have no option but to take extreme measures to change your outcomes. And when those extreme measures don't work, you can become frustrated and start feeling like your goals for weight loss and health are next to impossible. But I promise, it's not you. It's them! It's false promises and misinformation. These foods and extreme diets don't deliver. None of us ever really had a chance on them.

Reaching your goals through extreme behavior isn't just a problem in nutrition, of course. You'll see the same kind of promises made about exercise, too.

When I was brought in to train Halle Berry, Robert Downey, Jr., and Penélope Cruz for the movie *Gothika*, I had some explaining to do, especially with Halle, who was my main focus for the film.

At the beginning of our first session, Halle told me she was looking forward to working with me, but she had worked with the same trainer in L.A. for twelve years, and once she was done on set, she would be going back to him. We met for our first workout, which the studio booked at ninety minutes together. After twenty-five minutes, I told Halle we were done. She looked at me like I was crazy. *"What do you mean we're done? I need to get in great shape, and this won't get me in great shape. I work for ninety minutes."* I told her that we don't need ninety minutes. I explained that resistance exercise is like antibiotics. Sometimes taking extra doesn't necessarily help. Instead, it's about a specific frequency, duration, and intensity.

She didn't know what to make of it, but she didn't quit. The next session, she booked an hour. Again, we were done in twenty-five minutes. I could tell she was frustrated, but she came back again for a third session. When she showed up for that third workout, she didn't say much. Then, just as we were about to start, she gave me a big hug and told me her body felt like it never had before. She didn't know what had happened or what she was feeling, but she liked it. As they say, the rest is history. We worked together, and when she returned to L.A., I helped her prepare for *Catwoman*.

I remember one of the reviews for *Catwoman* saying that the movie was terrible, but at least her trainer did his job properly. Halle was in the best shape of her life, and she spent less time in the gym than ever.

NO FAT? ACTUALLY, NO GOOD.

In 1992, the food industry was about to change forever. That year, the USDA adopted the food pyramid for the first time (it had originated in Sweden in 1974). The 1992 pyramid recommendations were paired with the findings of a report—*Dietary Goals for the United States*—issued by the Senate Select Committee on Nutrition and Human Needs from fifteen years earlier. (No one ever said the government moves quickly.)

Those 1977 suggestions (issued via two reports) were actually pretty good. They recommended consuming less fat from saturated fats; eating more carbs from whole foods such as grains, legumes, fruits, and vegetables; and reducing added forms of salt and sugar in our diets. The problem is that the 1992 food pyramid oversimplified the guidelines, and the American public got the wrong message. More important, the recommendations probably didn't spend enough time emphasizing some of the finer details, and all the categories in the pyramid were left open to interpretation and manipulation.

The biggest misunderstanding about this food pyramid was right there at the top: that we should be eating fat, but sparingly. Eating *lower fat* is good, but too many people interpreted the new pyramid as

THE 1992 USDA FOOD PYRAMID

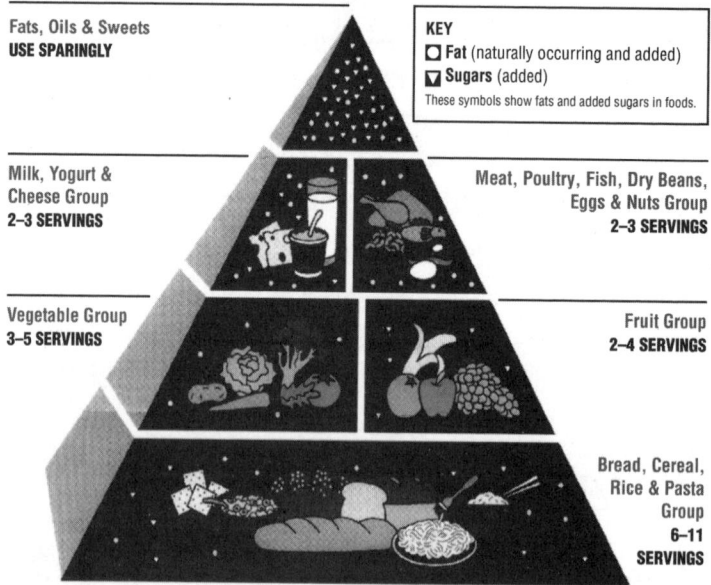

1992 USDA Food Guide Pyramid

recommending removing fat completely from the diet, which was *not* good. Healthy fat has many roles in your body, including helping with hormone production and brain function; cutting it out entirely is actually *unhealthy*.

But food manufacturers and marketers took this "no fat" idea and ran with it, focusing on less fat overall instead of less *saturated* fat. Big food companies became obsessed with low-fat everything. That meant changing the chemical structure of their products to make things taste irresistible (that is, replacing fats with a bunch of ingredients that are arguably less healthy but add to the taste). Our taste buds and cravings would never be the same. We were set on an endless spiral of labeling certain foods as bad and were encouraged to think of these manipulated, processed foods as better than nature's alternatives. You know what happened next: we all ate more of these "healthy" Frankenfoods than was actually good for us.

THE SNACKWELL'S EFFECT

Nothing highlighted this misinterpretation of the government-sanctioned dietary advice more than a line of cookies that was launched by Nabisco as a "healthy" choice: SnackWell's. They were just what the government ordered—very low in fat. But they were also loaded up with sugar to improve their taste. And they sold like mad.

The entire country seemed to fall under a low-fat spell (in truth it was more like mind control). We *all* fell for it. We didn't realize that we were replacing the fat with a massive amount of sugar because something had to be added to those processed foods to compensate for there being no fats in them; sugar made them taste good. But we know now that consuming all that sugar, not enough fiber and protein, and limited amounts of functional, healthy fats was a recipe for disaster.

Next thing you know, we were all consuming far too much sugar, making us crave more. A vicious cycle led to sugar being added to *almost everything,* transforming otherwise healthy foods—like bread and crackers, yogurt, and granola—into sneaky sources of weight gain. We were so worried about *any* amount of fat causing things like heart disease that we didn't grasp that one of the biggest drivers of those diseases wasn't fat as a macronutrient but overall *body fat.* We were made to believe that consuming fat made you fat, but the truth is to have less body fat, we need to eat fewer calories and consume more nutrient-dense foods. And to do *that,* we need fiber, but fiber wasn't a part of any of those high-sugar, fat-free treats.

What happened then was almost too predictable. As a society, we started gaining weight, obesity levels began to skyrocket, and we've been headed in the wrong direction ever since.

You would think the connection between rising obesity rates and the increased consumption of processed foods would have been obvious. Unfortunately, the opposite has been the case. We missed the forest for the trees. The Senate committee's guidelines recommended *less* saturated fat, *more* carbs, and *less* sugar and salt. It was *not* a sweeping moratorium on fat. The takeaway should have been, "Hey, some fat is good. Eat more avocados, nuts, and fatty fish. Eat a little less red meat, but you don't need to abandon it completely." Which is a perfectly reasonable plan that I can fully endorse—more on that later.

Instead, the food industry removed the saturated fat, pumped foods full of sugar and hydrogenated oils, and convinced us it was better for us.

Then, we started to wise up to just how much sugar we were eating in those "healthy" low-fat snacks, and we had a new villain. Don't get me wrong—too much sugar can definitely be an issue—but, in the all too predictable overcorrection, almost all carbohydrates were lumped into the same category as refined and added sugars. So, in an effort to reduce our sugar intake, we oversimplified again, this time vilifying carbs. But lost in the conversation was the fact that carbs contain vital nutrients, without which we yet again saw declining health, more weight gain, and enough frustration over trying to lose weight to last a lifetime.

That's the *real* lasting impact of SnackWell's and the trend of villainizing an entire food group. It wasn't the snacks themselves (as of 2022 they've been discontinued). It was the marketing plan, which ushered in a new age of how to sell "health" foods. And that game plan has been repeated by countless companies and led tens of millions of unsuspecting people toward foods that did more harm than good.

Why Losing Weight Can Feel Impossible
Have you ever
- tried a detox?
- done a cleanse?
- followed a zero-carb diet?
- cut out nightshades and legumes?
- stopped eating eggs or dairy?
- eaten only raw foods?
- avoided fruit (because they have sugar)?

No shame or blame here, but I'm going to bet that you may have answered yes to at least one of those questions. Don't beat yourself up.

You are not alone in having tried, and most likely failed at, some of these diet approaches.

Another important question: Have you ever lost weight on a diet only to gain back the weight—and then some—when you stopped dieting? Here again, I'm guessing the answer is yes and I'm sorry to say that's because you were misinformed. So much of how we diet reflects how marketers make you *perceive* the dangers of food. Every time a new piece of health information comes out, marketers take advantage of the new trend and then take an extreme approach in their messaging, which leads to an extreme change in our behaviors. See SnackWell's above!

If you are like most people, you try to "diet" because the numbers on the scale have hit a place that you don't like, you want to look better at an upcoming event, or beach season is around the corner. Most people diet as a quick fix for an issue, but diets don't need to be temporary. In fact, your diet—by definition—is the way you eat day after day. But in the modern world dieting has become a temporary sprint toward an unrealistic goal and includes a plan that might get short-term results but will steal your progress the minute you stop these unsustainable efforts.

People like to say "the body keeps score," and it's certainly true when it comes to what you eat. If you strip your body of vital nutrients or remove too many calories, your body will react; you'll lose weight. Eventually, however, it will counteract in ways you don't expect and won't like. The weight goes down, then up . . . and up . . . and up. Start another diet, and it goes down; stop the diet and then up . . . and up . . . and up. The initial loss makes it seem that the diet works, but it's really the result that matters. And the result is often more weight than when you started.

The more extreme the diet, the less likely it is to stick. So you try one diet after another, having a little success and then regaining weight when you (and your body) can't take the diet's extreme restrictions anymore.

Yo-yoing through these dramatic shifts chips away at your good health habits, fills you with false representations of what it looks and feels like to be healthy, and pushes you far away from what you truly desire. If you want to change your body and improve your health, the plans you follow shouldn't feel like punishment.

THE THREE BIG DIET MISTAKES— AND HOW TO AVOID THEM

I'll admit that over the years I've experimented with many diets, even those I know are not supported by science or rock-solid research. Sometimes it's fun to try something out. After all, you want to find what works for your body. Unfortunately, discovering the "you" solution has become more complicated than ever. Rather than embracing the unique nature of every individual body and focusing on big-picture goals (sleep, carbs, protein, fruits, and vegetables), the diet industry majors in the minor. It seems like you'll become healthier if you can just suffer through fringe, extreme behavior.

Guess what? It's all a lie.

There are a few roadblocks to health that I want you to try to avoid because they are likely the reason that you have struggled to lose weight in the past. By becoming aware of these common mistakes, you can take the next steps on the path to better health.

Diet Mistake #1: The Harder It Feels, the Better It Must Work

If you woke up one day and decided you wanted to lose weight, what would you do? You might start by throwing out all the remotely delicious food you have in your kitchen. You might fill your grocery cart with chicken, eggs, nuts, and asparagus—not a carb in sight. Never mind that you despise asparagus. You're on a mission and you've heard that eating asparagus is *the* way to lose weight.

For the first few days, you will probably feel strong as you ride the wave of your surge of motivation. You tell yourself, "I can do this!" But then the hunger hits, and soon the cravings sneak up on you, which leaves you thinking, *"There's no way I can keep doing this."*

Maybe you tough it out for a few more days or weeks. You smile to yourself because you think that as you suffer silently, your fat is melting away. You are making a sacrifice for your health, right? But there are limits to what you can do. When you change how you eat, particularly when you do so dramatically, there will be some starts and stops. At some point, your progress will stall. You'll then be forced to drop your calories further, and you're going to dip into dangerous territory.

Diet Mistake #2: The Faster, the Better

Along the same lines as the painful plans, we seem to have faith in diets that give us quick results. For many, it's likely that no amount of progress will feel fast enough. Down one pound in a week? Something must not be working. Three pounds? That's more like it—but maybe more should have dropped by now. Five? Not bad, but why not ten? If this describes your logic, I'm sorry to have to tell you that you've been completely deceived about what to expect from your body. A few years ago, I wrote a book called 5 Pounds. It got rave reviews from the medical community and dietitians across the globe but sold fewer copies than any of the many books I have written. In an attempt to understand why it essentially bombed, we did some market research and discovered that the title was a fail. The critical takeaway was that losing five pounds wasn't sensational enough (or aspirational enough). People want to lose five pounds in a week—it's not their ultimate goal. We were told by consumers they would have been excited to purchase a book called 50 Pounds, but not one called 5 Pounds. I think that this is a perfect example of what is wrong with any diet mentality. People are trying to hit grand slams rather than single after single, and in the process, most people are striking out entirely.

Here's the truth: barring any health complications, most people can expect to lose an average of one to two pounds per week. There may be some weeks where you might see weight loss of more than three pounds, but they are the exception to the rule. Leaner people can expect a slower rate of one-half to one pound per week because they have less fat to lose, while extremely overweight or obese people can likely lose weight at a faster rate.

Anything faster than what is outlined above indicates you are likely losing too much too fast, which means you're also losing *muscle* and not *fat*. The numbers on the scale might look good to you at first, but hunger will increase dramatically, your hormones will be affected, and it will become harder to stick to the plan. The rebound effect will cause you to yo-yo from one diet to another.

When you have realistic expectations, losing anywhere from five to ten pounds per month is an incredible accomplishment. It's when you assume that this amount of weight loss can occur over the course of ten days that you feel frustrated or disappointed. If you shift your expectations, you can begin to enjoy the process of changing how you eat (and enjoying it), as well as really appreciating the positive changes happening to your body right before your eyes.

Diet Mistake #3: Obsessing About Superfoods

Perhaps this has happened to you: You're scrolling through social media and next thing you know, you're two minutes into a video about a new superfood. At first, you're skeptical, but—at the same time—you *want* to believe there's an easier way to be healthier. Buzzwords jump off the screen like *metabolism, microbiome,* and *adaptogens.* All you have to do is fork over your money and the problems you haven't been able to solve in the past will be fixed right now. According to the sales pitch, you don't have to change your current lifestyle. All you need to do is sprinkle this amazing powder into your morning coffee, and you'll be good to go. No fuss, no muss. The truth is that none of these (typically very expensive) "superfoods" are the miracle solution the hype promises.

If you want superfoods that will make a positive difference in your diet, you don't need to shop at an expensive grocery store to find them. All you need are the tried-and-true, classic fruits and vegetables, as well as grains, legumes, and lean proteins that are filled with the body-transforming nutrients you desire.

Technically, you can lose weight on any diet. Some people consume a monotropic diet, aka eating only a single type of food all the time. I remember reading that the famous industrialist Howard Hughes would go for weeks eating nothing but canned soup. Other examples are health advocate Bernarr Macfadden, who in the 1920s created the milk-only diet that recommended twenty-eight cups of milk a day. In 2010, Chris Voigt ate twenty potatoes a day for two months and lost almost twenty pounds. A few years later, magician Penn Jillette also did the potato-only diet for two weeks and lost nearly twenty pounds as well. In no way am I advocating for this extreme type of diet, but it shows two things: you can lose weight for a short period of time following almost any diet and you can lose weight eating lots of carbs. But of all these extremes, my favorite was demonstrated by Dr. Mark Haub, a professor at Kansas State University. He decided to prove that dieting was about only how many calories you consume. He devised a plan: eat a famous dessert every day—and lots of it—and measure what happens. Haub lost twenty-seven pounds by eating mostly Twinkies.[3] This wasn't an attempt to sell "the Twinkie diet" or to tell people to follow a sugar-loaded eating plan. On a deeper level, he was demonstrating how you can manipulate calories and lose weight, even if you're not choosing the healthiest foods. As you can imagine, Twinkies are not the answer to losing weight any more than swearing off carbohydrates will do the trick. Living a healthy life requires change, some of which might feel difficult. But the changes should not make you think, *"Wow, that sounds crazy!"*

I understand it can be hard to determine if something sounds ridiculous when you're already frustrated by how you feel and you desperately want a change, so I've come up with a question to help you in your decision-making process.

Anytime you are considering a diet, ask yourself: *"Would I be comfortable feeding a child this way?"* It could be your own child, a niece or nephew, or the little ones of your closest friends. You can use the "child test" on any of the extreme diets that you've ever heard of. Would you ever be comfortable suggesting that they never eat fruits and vegetables? Would you cook them endless amounts of bacon, stuff it between two meat patties, and call it a healthy meal? What about the occasional treat? Is it healthy for them to stress and feel guilty about every ounce of sugar they consume? The answer to all of this is no. If you wouldn't feed your child in a certain way, you should consider applying similar rules to yourself. Otherwise, you risk damaging your body as well as your relationship with food.

The diet industry knows how to take advantage of your insecurities and the complicated nature of nutrition. You hear *Twinkie diet* and think of a gimmick. But, if a doctor sells you on the idea that "grains will destroy your brain," that feels more believable. The plausibility of this way of thinking makes it far more dangerous than the Twinkies.

> If you wouldn't feed your child in a certain way, you should consider applying similar rules to yourself. Otherwise, you risk damaging your body as well as your relationship with food.

You can control the way you eat and avoid extreme diets, and it can have a life-changing impact. I know because I've seen it happen repeatedly for people of all shapes, sizes, genders, and lifestyles.

Ironically, the more science has advanced, the more we have regressed in our ability to lose weight. Why? Probably because 99 percent of the diet industry is caught somewhere between self-experimentation and pseudoscience. It's the world's greatest (and worst) case study of science gone wrong. The good news is, we can turn it all around. Instead of focusing on the 1 percent of studies that suggest a "diamond in the rough" approach, it's more effective to search for the jewels where they are easiest to find. Discovering these jewels and putting them into action means relying on tips and tricks that are less flashy but more effective. Not to mention, that are much more enjoyable and sustainable.

THE REAL SECRETS OF HEALTHY PEOPLE

I understand the desire to make quick changes. In my line of work, I'm under pressure to deliver transformation for people on camera or on the stage. However, I don't promise the fastest results; I promise the best results. To my clients and to you. Furthermore, I promise you an outcome that will make you happily ditch the dieting cycle. When you're on the right path, you won't burn out, think your body is broken, or feel like a failure. You'll feel better, look better, and the positive changes will be something you can maintain.

The path I'm going to lead you on is not what you may imagine. First, healthy people have carbs in their diet. Healthy people don't work out in the gym for hours, and don't save their movement for workout time, but they move throughout the day. Healthy people go to bed earlier, don't drink much alcohol, and limit how much sugar they eat. But they also understand there's a time and place to bend those rules, stay up late, have a few drinks, and indulge. They understand they *don't* need to be perfect all the time, and that Sunday brunch is a great time for waffles, butter, and syrup—and any day can be brunch day—just not every day. You've been conditioned to believe that there's a time and a place to enjoy food, but I want to teach you how to make *all* meals enjoyable. And if you eat those waffles, there's no need to follow up with extreme behavior or punishment for your "indulgence." That's what nutrition should be like when you're on the right path. It's easier, more enjoyable, and gets results.

Often, we don't realize how these extreme diets corrode and infiltrate our day-to-day living. Healthy people have relationships, real "social networks," and people who bring them joy, emotional support, and motivation. These offline social networks limit the need for the online ones—that means healthy people don't sit and look at a screen ten or twelve hours a day. Healthy people stop looking for the one thing that solves a problem and start looking for all the things that make them feel good and build healthy habits around those things.

Real researchers don't spend time arguing about the single secret to weight loss. They investigate why we gain weight, why it's hard to keep it off, and the collateral damage of failed diets. Research suggests that a few dietary basics will help you upgrade your health, regardless of your dietary preferences. Whether you eat animals or prefer a vegan style of diet, drink dairy, or have allergies, the right diet is the one that avoids an extreme narrative and brings balance back to the way you eat.

You didn't gain weight in one day and you won't lose it immediately either—at least not in a way that will allow you to keep it off in the long term. After all, less than 20 percent of people keep off the weight for more than a year.[4]

Instead, it's far better to follow a diet that primarily (but not exclusively) consists of real foods (think carbs, proteins, fruits, vegetables, nuts, grains, and legumes), while also providing enough flexibility to eat some foods that you like. The only real "secret" to dieting is to find a plan that you can realistically follow for as long as possible—not just for four weeks or sixty days.

EAT, DON'T OVERTHINK

As discussed, many approaches to eating can result in weight loss. But you need to stop asking whether something works to change the numbers on the scale or whether something works in the best interest of your body and mind. When it comes to better eating for health, you need to put yourself back in the driver's seat and avoid the potholes and detours that can throw you off course.

STOP OVERCOMPENSATING

At some point, you're going to have a bad day (it's inevitable) and not follow your plan to a T. Maybe stress will get the best of you, you'll be overtired, or you'll have such an amazing night out with friends that all dietary guidelines fall by the wayside. These moments happen. And much like having small treats now and again, these moments can be just a blip on the radar of your overall healthy eating—but only if you *don't* make a big deal out of them. Successful weight loss and good health don't require 100 percent compliance. Instead, they require consistent commitment.

If you have an "off" day of eating, resist the urge to overcorrect or starve yourself. You don't need to do anything other than return to the normal plan. Don't fast. Don't juice. Don't detox. Just eat regularly, and your body will thank you.

GIVE UP ON METABOLISM HACKING

Everyone wants a faster metabolism. And there's no shortage of products and pills promising to help you burn more calories. They are all fool's gold.

With *The Carb Reset*, you'll be eating the foods that give you the best chance to maximize calorie burning. Don't invest time and money in things that are more likely to burn more money and patience than calories.

AVOID THE "HEALTH FOOD" MINDSET

There are lots of healthy foods that you should eat more often. I want you to embrace a mindset of abundance over one of restriction. But a common fallacy is that just because something is considered healthy, you can eat seemingly unlimited amounts of it. The laws of good health and fat loss are not the same.

If you eat too much of any food—even a nutritious option—it can lead to weight gain. For example, nuts and seeds are great. I want you to eat them on your path to a healthy weight, but they are also loaded with calories. If you eat too many nuts just because they are good for you, you can end up frustrated because eventually those calories will add up. Except for vegetables, there are limits on how much you can eat of any food. But don't worry about having to overthink this. When you follow the style of eating I detail in this book, you'll naturally feel full and give your body everything it needs.

STOP COUNTING CALORIES

It is true that if calories in exceed calories out you will gain weight, and if calories in are fewer than calories out, you will lose weight. However, this equation is not food dependent, meaning that x number of calories of ice cream and the same number of calories of fruit aren't processed the same way in your body. Counting calories "works," but doing so won't give you the freedom to eat the foods you like, keep balance in your diet, or make healthy food choices. Plus, obsessing over every calorie you eat is no fun.

DON'T WORRY ABOUT MEAL TIMING

The less you stress about food, the more you can enjoy eating it. This goes not only for the foods you eat but also *when* you eat. There are many myths about how much you can eat at each meal, whether you need to eat immediately after waking, or what you have to eat the moment a workout ends. The reality is that the timing of meals is very much overrated. What you eat and how much you eat determine how you feel as well as your results much more than trying to time each meal to the minute.

MEAL TIMING?

Scientific evidence suggests that meal timing is *not* a critical factor for weight loss or weight gain:

1. **TOTAL CALORIC INTAKE IS KEY:** Numerous studies, including a systematic review published in 2015, emphasize that *total daily* caloric intake is the primary influence on weight loss or gain, regardless of meal timing. As long as caloric balance (calories in versus calories out) is maintained, the timing of meals appears to have minimal impact on body composition changes.[5]

2. **MEAL TIMING AND METABOLISM:** A 2018 study assessed whether different meal timing schedules affected weight loss and metabolic markers. Findings indicated no significant differences in weight loss among groups with different meal timings, emphasizing that timing had minimal impact.[6]

3. **LONG-TERM STUDIES:** Longitudinal studies demonstrate that variations in meal frequency and timing do not consistently influence weight outcomes over extended periods. Factors such as following dietary guidelines and overall food quality are more strongly correlated with sustained weight management.[7]

4. **IMPACT ON PHYSICAL PERFORMANCE:** Studies suggest that while timing of eating in relation to workouts may influence performance and recovery, the timing of other meals throughout the day does not significantly affect body composition outcomes when total daily caloric and nutrient needs are met.[8]

5. **INDIVIDUAL VARIABILITY:** Recent research underscores the variability in metabolic responses to meal timing. Some people may experience slight differences in glucose and insulin responses based on meal timing, but these differences do not consistently contribute to significant changes in weight over time.[9]

While meal timing may influence factors like performance and metabolic responses in some people, the overall impact on weight loss or gain appears to be minimal when compared with the total caloric intake and nutritional quality of meals consumed throughout the day.

If it helps you to have a set meal schedule that doesn't cause anxiety, then do what works for you. Keep in mind, however, that there's no need to overemphasize having a meal at a specific time of day. Just follow the meal plans I've provided in chapter 10 and eat when it's convenient for you.

THE EXCEPTION TO THE FOOD RESTRICTION RULE: ALLERGIES AND INTOLERANCES

As strongly as I feel about each of us being able to be flexible and enjoy lots of foods on the path to losing weight and staying healthy, there are people for whom avoiding certain foods (or whole food categories) is a necessity. It goes without saying that if you have an allergy to a particular food, you should not eat it. It also makes good common sense to avoid eating foods if you have an intolerance. But what do you do if it's not so clear-cut? Time to do a little detective work.

The biochemistry of certain foods, meaning their chemical makeup, is most likely to blame for gastrointestinal issues, from mild cramps or slight nausea after eating to the more serious cramping and discomfort of irritable bowel syndrome (IBS). For example, some people can drink gallons of coffee with no issue, while one cup will send others sprinting for the bathroom. Those untroubled by coffee may have developed a tolerance from years of drinking it. And those who have an issue may have a body that is not chemically suited to handling the combination of salicylates (naturally occurring chemicals that often function as natural pest deterrents) and caffeine.

If you are not sure if a particular food is causing issues, you'll want to use an elimination process to single out the foods that may be causing gastrointestinal distress. An elimination diet is used as a diagnostic tool to see which foods you could be allergic to or have an intolerance for. You eliminate foods (over the course of a week or two) that can cause a reaction and reintroduce them, one at a time (over two or three days). If you experience gastrointestinal discomfort after the reintroduction, that's a sign that the food in question—the one you just tried to reintroduce—is problematic for you. Foods that commonly trigger an allergic reaction or intolerance (typically indicated by digestive issues) are peanuts, soy, eggs, milk, shellfish, citrus fruits, nightshade vegetables (tomatoes, potatoes, eggplants, bell peppers), and gluten (found in wheat, barley, and rye). (Note that there is a gluten-free swap list in chapter 10.)

If you have IBS, there is one restriction diet that has science on its side: the FODMAP diet. FODMAP stands for Fermentable Oligosaccharides, Disaccharides, Monosaccharides, and Polyols, a natural set of components in the foods you eat. Researchers studying irritable bowel syndrome have found that eliminating FODMAP foods is a reliable way to soothe GI distress and food intolerance. Any gastroenterologist or registered dietitian familiar with the low-FODMAP diet should be able to walk you through the basic eliminations.

At first, the cuts may seem severe (onions, garlic, and some veggies and fruits are on the list), but as I described above for the general process for elimination diets, after a few weeks, you can reintroduce one food at a time. If you have a reaction, you'll know which food you struggle to digest.

To get you started, here is a list of foods that you might want to consider removing if you have stomach discomfort.

- **Fermentable Oligosaccharides:** barley, chicory, garlic, legumes, lentils, onions, wheat, rye
- **Disaccharides:** dairy products containing lactose, such as ice cream, milk, or yogurt
- **Monosaccharides:** apples, mangoes, pears, watermelons
- **Polyols:** apricots, cauliflowers, plums, and many artificial sweeteners (maltitol, mannitol, sorbitol, xylitol)

Split up the foods into groups of three to five foods so that you don't tackle too many foods at once. After three weeks without the foods, add one food back in at a time for three or four days. See if you have a reaction. If not, that food isn't the issue, and you can continue building your diet back with freedom and comfort.

Next, let's look at my PATH approach to resetting your plate, resetting your relationship with carbs, and getting you on the road to better health.

CHAPTER 2

PATH:
An Eating Plan That Fits
in the Palm of Your Hand

I advocate eating from all the food groups and don't waste time demonizing one food over another. This doesn't mean that you can eat whatever you want, whenever you want, but the goal is to have balance on your plate. *The Carb Reset* works by using the PATH acronym to guide your food choices.

As you've learned, many plans are obsessed with fat burning and completely ignore fat storage. But eating foods that minimize fat storage—which also tends to mean eating foods with lower energy density that are more filling and fuel your entire body—can deliver much better results.

So much dietary frustration stems from the fact that most diets are so rigid that it feels impossible to personalize them. Uniquely, the proportions of macronutrients represented by the PATH acronym are inspired by scientifically supported, well-established diets from around the globe. These cuisines have gotten it right and provide a foundation for helping you stay healthy in the long run, without feeling deprived.

The Japanese diet, for example, has stood the test of time. It's the dietary plan followed by one of the longest-living populations in the world, which also happens to be one of the biggest consumers of carbohydrates. The diet is built around rice, but it's also filled with fish and eggs, vegetables, and pickled foods. Despite being high in carbohydrates, it's also low in sugar.

Another cuisine I draw from is the Scandinavian diet. It features fish and lean protein but, instead of focusing on rice as in Japan, it has carbs like whole grains, rye, barley, and amazing bread and crackers. It also includes high-protein forms of dairy like yogurt, and in particular Skyr.

Of course, there's also the much-written-about and -lauded Mediterranean diet, which focuses on whole grains and olive oil, lentils and legumes, berries and citrus, seafood, eggs, dairy, and a variety of nuts and seeds.

I've taken the best of all these worlds and am bringing it to your table to provide balance in the form of a PALM of carbohydrates, ALL the vegetables you want to eat, a THUMB of healthy fat (while limiting saturated fats and excess oils), and a HAND of protein at every meal. Put it together and this life-changing eating program features:

- More fiber
- Plenty of fruits and vegetables
- Moderate protein, from a variety of sources
- Limited saturated fats
- A good dose of healthy, unsaturated fats
- Lower sugar (but no need to go zero sugar)
- Lots of variety and flavor

You get to choose—rice, whole grains or buckwheat, rye or barley, wheat or legumes, or fermented carbs such as sourdough bread. You don't need to eat all these carbs; you simply need to find the ones you enjoy and make them a part of your daily meals. You also get to balance out the carbs with the protein of your choice, and that can come from meat, fish, or plant-based sources. The healthiest, longest-living populations in the world eat this way and have the lowest incidence of diabetes, heart disease, and most cancers. These diets, and my approach, don't go to extremes. That's the real secret of a life-changing diet. They don't recommend exclusively eating meat or suggest you need to be completely plant-based or vegan. They include more plants, but not to the exclusion of other foods. They embrace carbs from grains. They don't fear protein. And they don't feature ultraprocessed packaged foods that can have copious amounts of added sugar.

The one thing all these dietary approaches have in common is they don't feature a lot of beef or lamb—which can be high in fat. Lean cuts of these red meats are okay, but most protein comes from other sources, whether it's fish, dairy, legumes, or eggs, as well as some poultry and maybe a little pork. You'll learn more about your healthiest options for meats in chapter 6.

The Carb Reset is filled with foods you can find in any store, can cater to any personal preferences, and will benefit every aspect of your health. You'll stay fuller for longer, not fall for the same traps of other diets that fail, and you'll finally eat in a way that you not only enjoy but helps you lose weight at the same time.

You've probably never allowed yourself to consume a carb-based diet before (at least a low-sugar carbohydrate diet like this one). While it may seem almost too simple, I am here to tell you that it is the most effective at meaningful and long-term weight management. After they try it, most people I work with never want to eat any other way again. It's fun because you have lots of options, there are choices that give you flavor and variety, and you aren't limited to only a few foods— essentially, there are endless ways of making it work.

One of the keys to achieving the right balance in this diet is eating the *right* carbohydrates, because there is a continuum of options you should eat more often and those you should enjoy less frequently. The carbohydrates you can consume in relatively limitless amounts include options like vegetables. The carbs that you should have less frequently are sweets and baked goods. When you feed your body the right way, it can handle moderate amounts of sugar. Back in university, we were told you should minimize certain fats (like saturated fats found in red meat) and enjoy other healthier options (like monounsaturated fats found in avocados and nuts). We were always told that whole foods was the best way to go. So, eat an orange, skip the orange juice; enjoy rice, but not rice flour; and eat quinoa and not quinoa crackers. You'll learn more about all these specifics in the coming chapters devoted to each of the macronutrient components of my PATH strategy.

I often have to convince clients that walking is at least as effective, if not more effective, for weight loss when compared with running or sprinting or spinning. People think they need to exercise with the highest intensity possible to achieve the greatest weight loss. If I asked two people to go five miles and one person sprinted as fast as they could and the other walked, the person sprinting would get farther faster, but most likely would burn out and not make it the entire five miles. The person moving at a sensible, moderate walking pace would pass their sprinting counterpart and most likely have no problem making it to their five-mile goal. The same is true when it comes to diet. Eating in an extreme way might initially get you further faster (that is, you'll lose weight quickly), but you will never reach your goal—and reaching your goal is the point, right?

Once you learn how to follow the PATH, I think you'll see it's much easier to create that balance on your plate.

NEVER STRESS CALORIES AGAIN

It has been said that the way to achieve weight loss is adhering to the calories-in versus calories-out model, so by eating fewer calories than you burn you can lose weight. From a thermodynamics standpoint, this is accurate. From a lifestyle standpoint, it's not quite that simple. If you take two identical people and one of them eats 1,500 calories a day of broccoli, salmon, and avocado, and the other consumes 1,500 calories a day of processed snacks and sugary liquids (soda and the like), and even if they engage in the same amount of movement/calorie burning, over time those two people will not look the same. Assuming they have the same calorie output through their physical activity, they will actually lose the same amount of weight in the short term. However, over time, their body compositions and health will diverge. The foods you eat influence how your body functions, from the way your hormones react, to the energy you have for exercising, to how well you sleep, as well as the way your metabolism functions overall.

That doesn't mean calories in and calories out doesn't work, and that you shouldn't consider calories when you are eating, but I want you to focus on the *composition* of your diet and the actual foods you are eating—rather than the calories you take in and the calories you burn—and make sure you're eating the right foods in the right amounts. The rest will take care of itself.

THE PATH APPROACH

The PATH approach is a simple way to think about eating, and will give your body all that it needs, without your having to stress about calories, weigh your foods, or worry if you're getting enough of the good stuff to support your body's needs. It's an acronym to help you remember what to put into each meal. Every time you grab a plate, I want you to think about being on the right PATH to better health, having more energy, and finding joy and freedom in your meals.

PATH STANDS FOR

Palm of carbohydrates

All the vegetables

Thumb of fat (from the base of your thumb on the palm side)

Hand of protein (it's the mass of your hand—whether rolled up into a fist or with your fingers extended)

If you follow these guidelines, you'll be eating in a way to help you to lose weight, be healthier, increase energy, and have the body you want. It simplifies how you choose the amounts of what you need to eat, because all you need is your hand to measure your portions—it's a diet that fits in your hand!

PATH FLEXIBILITY

This plan is so successful because of its flexibility—there are no hard rules about what you can and can't eat. Granted, there are some foods that you can eat more often and others that you will eat sparingly, but these are guidelines, not make it or break it rules. The days of whole food groups being completely off-limits are over—remember my cookie that I eat every day? The PATH plan includes *all* the food groups, so you never have to stress about keeping particular foods off your plate. And to repeat—and because so many people are astonished to hear it these days—carbs, one of the first things to be eliminated from most diets, form the cornerstone of PATH.

The PATH plan is based on a massive body of research that clearly demonstrates the long-term effectiveness of having more carbs in your diet. In a yearlong, randomized clinical trial (DIETFITS), scientists found that a healthy low-fat diet versus a healthy low-carbohydrate diet produced similar weight loss and improvements in metabolic health markers.[1]

The researchers also found that insulin production—the hormone released by eating carbs—had no impact on predicting weight-loss success or failure. In other words: eating more carbs is *not* the cause of weight gain. But it's not just that weight loss was the same. It's that the people who eat more carbs had an easier time following and sticking to the plan.

In a world of overcomplicated meal plans and stress-inducing rules about the timing of meals, there's something incredibly powerful about simplicity. My plan is super easy to remember, and that alone can help it be effective. It is something you can sustainably follow over a long period of time. In fact, you can follow it for the rest of your life. The more your body becomes used to eating carbs—rather than yo-yoing between eating carbs and banishing them from your diet—the better you will process them, the less you will bloat, and the easier it will be to transform your health and your body.

HOW IT WORKS

The PATH approach is designed to help your body use the right carbs (less fat storage) at the right times in every meal to help you feel satisfied, cut cravings, and keep your body losing weight without your having to overthink anything. At each meal, you'll be able to enjoy carbohydrates, protein, and fat, along with plenty of nutritious vegetables. It's the true definition of balance and moderation, without your having to overthink everything you put into your body.

CARBS

For your starchy carbs, a serving size fills your **palm**. This applies to foods like rice, pasta, or cut-up fruits. When it comes to single servings—like sliced bread or a whole fruit—one slice of high-fiber bread (more than 3 grams per serving) or one medium piece of fruit works. Either way, this will be approximately 1 cup.

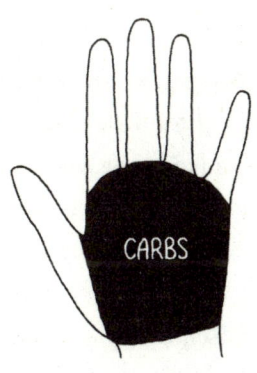

VEGGIES

"A" STANDS FOR ALL THE VEGGIES

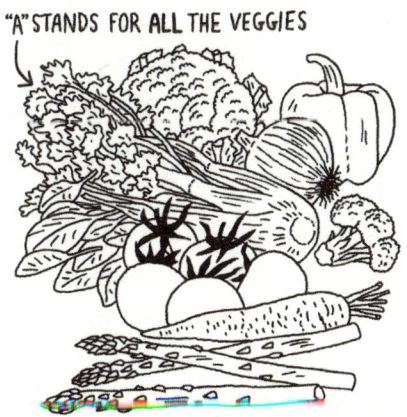

You should feel free to have **all** the vegetables—as many vegetables as you want—whether it's leafy greens, tomatoes, bell peppers, or asparagus—you name it. Sneak those veggies into sandwiches, blend them into soups and smoothies, cook them with your eggs, or sauté them to add to pasta.

If you love veggies, that's great! If you don't, I'm not going to convince you how delicious they are, but I am confident that you will enjoy the meals, including vegetables, that you will create on this program.

FATS

For fats, simply measure the amount that matches the approximate distance from the tip of your **thumb** to its base. This applies to oils you'll use in cooking or add to salads, or for foods like avocados, nuts, nut butters, seeds, and hummus. For liquids (like oils), this is about 1 tablespoon; for solids (like avocado), it's approximately 1 ounce.

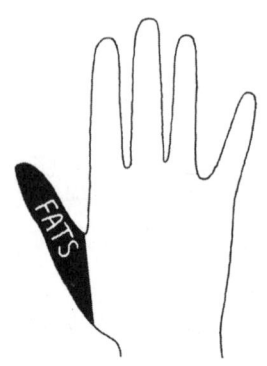

PROTEIN

Protein is the most metabolic food, it helps you feel full, and it's the most difficult to store as fat in your body. This applies to all protein options, whether it's chicken or fish, or plant-based sources like tofu or black beans.

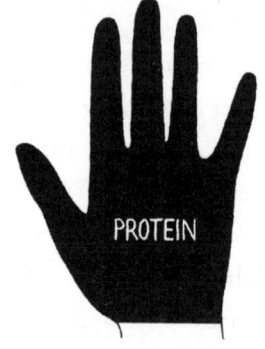

A serving size of protein should be equal to the mass of your entire **hand**, including your fingers. For most people, that amounts to 4 to 6 ounces. However, larger people might have higher requirements; that is, more than 4 to 6 ounces. Protein requirements are based on body weight (to some extent). For example, the government suggests 0.8 gram of protein per kilogram of body weight per day—however, there is some research that indicates as much as 1.8 grams of protein per kilogram of body weight per day may be effective. Personally, I like to hit smack-dab in the middle at about 1.5 grams of protein per kilogram of body weight per day. For the most part, a 100-kilogram person (about 220 pounds) is going to have a bigger hand than a 60-kilogram person, and because protein requirements are based on body weight—to a degree—a larger person will have a larger hand and have a larger serving of protein.

Remember, this way of eating doesn't limit the number or types of foods you consume. It helps you make choices about how to build a healthy meal that will make food work for your body, giving you freedom to choose the options you like from a range of food groups and nutrients. As I mentioned previously, there really aren't many bad foods. There are just bad meals and bad diets. And, when I say "bad diet," I mean a deprivation-based eating "plan" that has you 100 percent avoid eating complete food groups, makes you feel deprived (and often sad), and ultimately works against your body rather than with it. Bad diets are unsustainable, and once you inevitably quit one, you will likely gain back any weight you lost—and then some.

When I talk about following a diet, I mean adopting a few easy, accessible, and sustainable eating principles. This way of eating puts you in control by eliminating the restrictions you experience on a typical diet and giving you a visual way to guide your meals. It's grounded in science and is sustainable, healthy, and—most important—fun. You can eat this way for the rest of your life and never look back.

This approach makes it super simple to know what to eat—which is almost anything. The beauty is that you have almost limitless options that can fit into any meal. You *don't have* to eat fruits or vegetables at every single meal. You *don't need* to stress about a single source of protein or fat. You can simply balance your plate by using PATH, so you can eat, enjoy, and watch your body transform.

THE FOOD LIST

Not sure what to eat? Pick any of the foods below to build a meal that will work. This is not an exhaustive list, but it gives you a good idea of how you can put your meals together. Don't forget that in chapters 10 and 11, you'll find some sample meal plans and recipes as well.

PROTEIN	FATS	CARBOHYDRATES	VEGETABLES	FRUITS
Chicken (skinless breasts or thighs)	Olive oil	Sweet potatoes/ Yams	Any green leafy vegetable	Grapefruits
	Nuts (almonds, cashews, Brazil nuts)	Rice	Broccoli	Apples
Eggs (3:1 ratio of whites to yolks)		Beans	Spinach	Berries (strawberries, blackberries, raspberries, blueberries)
	Nut butters	Whole grains (quinoa, farro, amaranth, millet, barley, teff)	Arugula	
Beef (lean ground or cuts)	Avocados		Romaine	
	Egg yolks	Oats	Brussels sprouts	Watermelons
Pork tenderloin	Seeds (chia, flax)	High-fiber bread/ wrap	Asparagus	Bananas
		High-fiber pasta	Green beans	Oranges
Turkey (lean ground or skinless breasts)			Squash	Jicama
			Kale	
Greek yogurt			Tomatoes	
			Celery	
Nonfat cottage cheese			Zucchini	
			Carrots	
Whey, casein, egg white, or plant-based protein powder			Cucumbers	
			Cauliflowers	
			Eggplants	
Fish and seafood			Peas	
			Bell peppers	
Tofu				

EAT, DON'T THINK

Some people may look at these foods and wonder, "There are so many options, what should I eat?" Eating this way is an adjustment to what you are used to, so I've prepared sample meal plans, as well as meal templates, in chapter 10. Consider those as training wheels to help you adapt to this new, balanced way of eating. The beauty of the system is that you won't need those training wheels for long. Soon, you'll be able to select foods from these categories, measure quantities with your hand using the PATH guidelines, fill your plate, and all that is left to do is enjoy your meal. No more calorie counting, food weighing, or going to such extremes as keeping track of your blood sugar fluctuations after each meal.

You'll naturally be eating less sugar and saturated fat and giving your gut health the prebiotic nutrients it needs to be healthier. Eating by using the PATH guidelines is easily adaptable to your specific tastes, preferences, and needs.

CHAPTER 3

Skinny People Eat Bread
(and Other Delicious Carbs)

P = A PALM OF CARBOHYDRATES

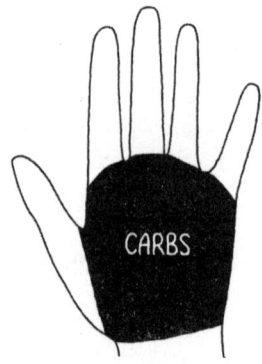

As is obvious from the title of this book, I feel strongly that we need to reset our relationship with carbs. That's why carbs are the first macronutrient I want to discuss and why—in the PATH acronym—I am encouraging you to have a palm(*P*)-size portion of them at every meal.

You've been told that enjoying rice, pasta, or other carbs is wrong, will make you fat, and will lead to a host of health issues. And yet research suggests that people who make room for those carbs on their plates and in their diets are doing something right. To understand why you've been misled, and that skinny people really do eat bread and pasta, it's important to realize that much of what you've been told about most of your carb-loaded foods simply isn't true. You can eat carbs and be healthy. I'll say that again: you can eat carbs and be healthy.

The idea that cutting carbs is the magic bullet for weight loss isn't new—we've been doing it since *Dr. Atkins' Diet Revolution* was published in 1972.* What is new is that for the last twenty years, we've been reducing our carb intake, and during that same time, the prevalence of obesity has continued to rise.

The mindset that no-carb plans are the *only* solution for losing weight has pushed people toward dietary behaviors that have been detrimental to overall health and, at the end of the day, sabotaged weight-loss goals.

Most carbs are not inherently more fattening or detrimental to your diet than other nutrients. The problem is that too often we think of sugary items like cakes, cookies, and sweetened breads as the only carbs out there. This discounts the powerfully good properties of a long list of "good carbs," which we'll get to momentarily.

First, we need to rewrite the story about carbs and engineer a reset to get you back on track. That starts by understanding why "cutting carbs" is a misleading solution and doesn't work the way you might think.

KETOGENIC DIETS: TAKING CARB CUTTING TO EXTREMES

When your body is in a "ketogenic state," it starts burning fat first for its needed fuel. That's the very broad-strokes logic to the ketogenic (or keto, for short) diets that are so popular these days. These diets have actually been around for a long time—as early as the late 1960s (when a diet known as the Stillman diet was popular). But when you examine the science behind them, you'll find that ketogenic diets are *not* more effective than other diets at burning fat.

---

* In fact, in the late 1700s, John Rollo was the first in the medical annals to promote a meat-only diet. However, it should be noted that this diet was developed for people with diabetes and before the discovery of insulin. Rollo did not promote it as a way to be healthy but only to help diabetics avoid blood sugar accumulation.

To put your body into a ketogenic state, you need to remove almost all carbs, start eating *a lot* of fat, and consume a moderate amount of protein. When you do this, your liver is forced to convert fat into fatty acids and ketones to give you energy. That's called being in ketosis, and—as I said above—is the point at which your body starts burning fat for its needed fuel. But this doesn't mean you are melting fat off the places you'd like to see it disappear—your stomach or thighs, for example—but rather you are burning the fat you eat, nothing more, nothing less.

Through ketosis, your body becomes what many call fat-adapted, meaning your body adjusts to what you're consuming and uses fat for energy. Unfortunately, becoming fat-adapted leads to feeling extreme fatigue, brain fog, and sluggish performance. Because your brain is the primary user of your body's carbs and a substance called glucose (carbs converted into energy), when you don't have that fuel, your entire central nervous system feels the negative effects.

Another way of looking at it is this: The "energy" your body needs is glucose. In the absence of carbs, because your body likes efficiency, it can make glycogen without carbs, but the energy doesn't come from stored fat—it comes from muscle (a process called gluconeogenesis). Your muscle that is now being used for fuel was intended to support a healthy, functioning metabolism, fight against aging, and make it easy for you to enjoy and process carbs.

So you can cut carbs and lose weight on a ketogenic diet, but it comes at a great cost. The numbers on the scale drop, but it's not necessarily due to loss of body fat; instead, you're losing muscle. This is how people can become "skinny fat." You lose weight, but your body doesn't look or feel the way you want. It's not inevitable, but it is the experience of most people who take the traditional "extreme restriction" dieting approach.

In fact, studies show that if you eat the same amount of protein on a low-carb diet as on a high-carb diet, there's no difference in fat burning; interestingly, eating more carbs might mean you consume *fewer* calories. When it comes to eating carbs versus fats, eating carbs can also lead to consuming fewer calories. Carbs fill you up, so by eating more carbs, which contain only 4 calories per gram, there is less room for consuming fat, which contains 9 calories per gram. The question is simple: *Do you want to work with your body or against it?* Once you realize that eating carbohydrates works *with* your body's natural preference, it opens up a new world of possibilities for the foods you can enjoy eating while at the same time losing fat, feeling better, and not creating a stressful relationship with food.

THE COST OF CUTTING CARBS

We saw that over the last thirty years, American carb intake has gone from 57 percent to 48 percent daily caloric intake, and health in the United States has declined. Compare that with countries like Japan, where people eat about 58 percent carbs and yet there is less obesity, improved longevity, and better overall health. Of course, this is not a direct cause-and-effect situation, but the relationship between more carbs and better health is hard to ignore. If you struggle with sleep, don't seem to have energy, and battle hunger and the scale, adding carbs could allow your hormones to start working with you and supporting great health.

Let's look more closely at the consequences of going low carb.

WEIGHT-LOSS FRUSTRATION

When you first start cutting carbs, you'll generally lose weight quickly. You may assume that you are losing body fat, but some of that "weight loss" will be loss of muscle mass. Additionally, a lot of that "weight loss" will be water weight. Carbs hold water, which is good for you because your body is primarily made of water, and being hydrated helps you function. As you cut carbs, there is less water in your cells and the numbers on the scale drop. It is easy to buy into the illusion that carbs make you fat because the moment you eat some delicious bread, you feel bloated and the number on the scale increases. It seems like a clear connection, but it wasn't the bread—it was your water-depleted state that made you seem to have lost and then gained. If you consistently incorporate carbs into your diet, one more or less piece of bread won't lead to bloating or weight fluctuations. The yo-yo effect of your weight going up and down can stop if carbs play a role in your daily food intake.

EXERCISE PERFORMANCE

Carbs are your body's preferred energy store. Most of us need carbohydrates to feel, function, and perform our best. Carbs load up your glycogen, which allows you to lift weights, go for runs and walks, or perform your favorite activities and sports. When you cut carbs too low, it is more difficult to push yourself and exercise. Research shows that as you drop carb intake, the rate of perceived exertion (RPE) directly increases, making exercise feel more difficult and less enjoyable. For most people, it's hard enough to have the motivation to work out. You don't need to make it even harder to exercise on an empty tank.

HORMONAL HELL

While the number of calories you eat ultimately determines whether you gain weight, your hormones control everything from your hunger and your metabolism to the way you store fat. When you cut carbohydrates, you could cause several issues with your hormones.

One hormone that is negatively impacted by low-carb diets is T3, a thyroid hormone that helps with the fat-burning process and helps manage blood sugar. When you drop calories and carbohydrates too low, your T3 levels also drop. The more you cut carbs, the more T3 levels decrease, affecting your ability to lose weight, have energy, and protect your overall health. It's easy to reverse the reduction in T3. When you start eating more carbs, T3 levels rise, and your body functions more naturally.

Low-carbohydrate or -calorie consumption has also been shown to suppress your levels of leptin. Leptin is a hormone released by the fat cells and helps the body maintain its weight by inhibiting hunger and regulating energy balance. For this reason, it is sometimes referred to as the "satiety" or "fullness" hormone.[1]

Cortisol is another important hormone in your body that helps to regulate your metabolism. When cortisol is at an optimum level, it's trouble for fat gain *and* fat storage. In other words, if you don't control cortisol, it becomes much harder to burn fat and control your hunger. Research suggests that your cortisol levels rise when you exercise and follow a low-carb diet.[2] This has a domino effect. Not only is it harder to lose fat but it's also harder to exercise effectively. In one study, half of the people eating the carb-deficient, protein/fat-rich diet couldn't complete the exercise program, whereas everyone in the carbohydrate group was able to finish the exercises.

Lower carbs not only impact your hormones and your ability to drop weight, but a deficiency in carbs can also be disruptive to your overall health, especially for women. Evolutionary research suggests that women are more sensitive to lower carb intakes. Your hypothalamus and pituitary glands work with your adrenal glands in something known as the HPA axis, which requires carbs. Women who don't have enough carbs can suffer from hypothalamic amenorrhea, which means your hormones get disrupted, and your levels of the reproductive hormones—FSH (follicle-stimulating hormone), LH (luteinizing hormone), estrogen, testosterone, and progesterone—all drop. In other words, it's a nightmare hormonal cocktail that will have an effect on everything from your immune system and mood to your energy level and metabolism. Result: you might store more body fat, your fertility may decrease, bone loss may increase, your sleep may be disrupted, and you may be more prone to mental health issues like depression.

DECREASED FRUIT CONSUMPTION

Fruits are carbohydrates. Whether intentional or not, the condemnation of carbs leads to people eating less fruit. Over the last ten years, there has been a nearly 20 percent decrease in fruit consumption in the United States. Indeed, in 2019, the CDC estimated that approximately one out of every ten Americans eats the minimum amount of recommended fruit.[3]

Perhaps people are wary of the natural sugar in fruit, but the reality is that less fruit in your diet can lead to more weight gain. Research published in *Nutrients* found that fruit has anti-obesity effects, and in a study of more than five thousand people, those who ate one serving of fruit per day were 10 percent less likely to be obese or overweight. Not to mention, Australian researchers found a strong link between fruit consumption and a decrease in stress for adults of all ages.

FEAR OF WHOLE GRAINS

Because of the inaccurate belief that our paleo ancestors didn't eat starchy carbs (and a surge in the gluten-free movement), almost every fiber-based carb has been kicked to the curb. But a 2021 review of more than seventy studies found that whole grains and starchy carbs are essential to maintaining a lower weight and reducing the likelihood of everything from diabetes to heart disease and cardiac events.[4]

That's because fiber plays a big role in keeping you fuller for longer. According to research published in *Clinical Nutrition*, people who kept bread (a great source of fiber) in their diet lost just as much weight as those who cut it out—but those who ate bread were better at sticking to their diets.[5]

DEVELOPING EXTREME DIET BEHAVIORS

The most damaging consequence of the low-carb movement has been that its very restrictive nature makes it unsustainable, creating a damaging relationship with food and possibly leading to yo-yo dieting.

It would be one thing if it were necessary to remove carbs to lose fat, but again, researchers have shown that lower-carb and higher-carb diets are equally effective for fat loss. But here comes the fine print:

most people on the low-carb diets were not able to sustain the plans for more than six weeks, whereas people who kept carbs in their diet could stick to a diet plan for a year and ultimately have better outcomes.

THE EIGHT BIG BENEFITS OF CARBS

It becomes easier to stop avoiding carbs entirely once you understand how they are essential to feeling good, performing well, and living your best life. If the science above about carbs and weight loss isn't convincing, here are eight reasons it's so essential for you to add more carbs to your diet.

1. CARBS FUEL YOUR BRAIN

Proponents of intermittent fasting suggest that limiting food is a way to increase mental clarity, but that's not how your brain works. Your brain works all day long, even when you sleep. It's the control system for your body. Your brain needs glucose to function optimally, but, unlike other cells in your body, your brain cells don't have the room to store much glucose and need to have a consistent supply. This doesn't mean you need to eat around the clock; it means you need enough carbs (that will convert to glucose through digestion) to help power your system. When you don't eat enough carbs, it's common to suffer from brain fog, have memory troubles, struggle to learn, or have difficulty with focus.

You know that feeling when you're *hangry* and irritable? That's a sign of not having enough carb fuel. Eat the right carbs, have them with each meal, and your brain (and mood) will thank you.

2. CARBS ARE THE HAPPINESS FOOD

Most people I know tend to be happier when they're eating carbs. It's not just because we all love pasta or a bowl of cereal. When you savor and enjoy your foods, the enzymes in your saliva break down complex carbs into simple sugars that your body can use as instant energy or store as energy for a later time. When carbs are consumed with protein, the synergy that involves an amino acid called L-tryptophan can boost serotonin production—the body's happy hormone. When serotonin levels are low, you can feel anxious, stressed, and unhappy, which can happen if you carb-starve your body. To keep serotonin at an optimum level you need to fuel your body with fiber-loaded foods like fruits, legumes, and whole grains, which will leave you feeling happier.

3. CARBS IMPROVE SLEEP

Tryptophan and serotonin aren't good only for putting a smile on your face. They also help to improve your sleep, and the tryptophan you get from carbs can be especially helpful.

Tryptophan is a building block for both serotonin and melatonin. Serotonin influences sleep, mood, and appetite. Melatonin promotes a regular sleep/wake cycle. Studies show that people with diets high in carbs fall asleep more quickly than people on low-carb diets—especially when carbs are consumed at dinner. The caveat is that these carbs should be complex whole carbs—that is, whole grains, tubers, and vegetables rather than refined or sugar-laden carbs. In fact, studies have shown increased rates of insomnia in people who consume high amounts of refined sugars in the hours before sleep. So consuming a high-carb diet, especially later in the day, can increase these beneficial chemicals in your brain and make you feel sleepy. Interestingly, some research has found that carbs such as kiwis and cherries, in particular, might help sleep.

4. CARBS PROTECT YOUR HEART

There is truth in that old saying "An apple a day keeps the doctor away." Apples are carbs, people! The magic of apples is tied to their nutrient density, specifically, how they are loaded with soluble fiber. This fiber, also found in oats, beans, and berries, dissolves in water and essentially forms a gel in your digestive tract that slows down digestion. It helps manage your blood sugar and lower your LDL ("bad") cholesterol, protecting your arteries and heart from plaque buildup and disease and plays a major role in heart health. The less sugar in your blood and the lower your LDL, the healthier your heart will stay and function.

5. Carbs Boost Gut Health

Over the last decade, one of the biggest breakthroughs in health has been the understanding that the amount and variety of microorganisms in your gut play a vital role in your overall health. While we're still learning so much about the power of probiotics and the microbiome (the helpful bacteria that aid digestion), the immune system, and more, we already know a great deal about the need for and the benefits of prebiotics.

Prebiotics are complex carbohydrates that feed your body in a way that helps your body naturally produce more of the probiotics—beneficial bacteria—it needs to support your gut health. In other words, instead of taking a bunch of supplements that your body might not be able to use, eating prebiotics (from carbs) supports your natural production of healthy bacteria that not only aid digestion but promote overall health. Prebiotic foods include asparagus, beets, Jerusalem artichokes, wheat, honey, bananas, barley, tomatoes, rye, peas, beans, and seaweed.

6. Carbs Aid Healthy Digestion

Some of the common side effects of low-carb diets are bloating, constipation, and stomach pain. No one enjoys feeling like this, no matter how many pounds you are losing. Some think that these GI issues are the result of eating more protein and fat. The true cause, however, is the absence of carbs in the diet. Just as we mentioned with heart health, weight loss, and gut health, the digestive system also needs the fiber that is provided by carbohydrates to function well. The combination of soluble and insoluble fiber you can get from carbs keeps you regular; it removes waste that can build up in your digestive system.

7. Carbs Power Your Workouts (and Recovery)

Finding the motivation to work out can sometimes be hard enough, so you don't need to make your life more difficult by not having the energy you need to exercise. When you follow *The Carb Reset,* you won't need to worry about having enough time to exercise. Everything I design for my clients is built around *not* needing hours to exercise. You need just a little bit of time to move and increase your heart rate. Being fueled by carbs will make sure your body has the energy it needs to support muscle function as well as reap the benefits of your workouts.

From your muscles to your brain and heart, good carbs are your body's preferred energy source. Carbs are stored as glycogen, which is essential for producing adenosine triphosphate (ATP), your body's primary energy source for exercise. Without carbs, your workouts can feel like a struggle. With them, you'll be able to push harder—and recover more quickly and efficiently.

8. Carbs Fuel Weight Loss

And, finally, we come back to weight loss, which is likely the reason you picked up this book in the first place.

The real power of the role of carbs in weight management is tied to carbs' ability to keep you feeling fuller for longer while still eating the foods you love. Bread, pasta, cereal, and many other "convenience" foods are loaded with carbs. Cutting them out can be difficult and is, in fact, completely unnecessary. The right carbs are filled with fiber, which—as you just found out—protects your heart and reduces "bad" cholesterol.

It also helps you keep the weight off as you lose. One of the most challenging aspects of weight loss is that when the numbers on the scale start to go down, you tend to feel hungrier. The more you lose, the hungrier you seem to get. This phenomenon may be why many people end up losing weight and then gaining it back. To counter this tendency is simple—eat foods that make you feel full. The fiber from healthy carbohydrates signals your brain to turn off your hunger cues and keep you satisfied. When you combine fiber-rich carbs with protein and fat, you have the perfect combination that will allow you to drop pounds without the crazy cravings. When you cut out the carbs, you're missing a central ingredient needed to manage your appetite. Plus, with carbs on board, you store less fat.

BURNING FAT VERSUS STORING FAT—
THE CARB CONNECTION

When my clients come to me, they want to lose weight or get in movie or TV-screen shape. You may not be preparing for stage or screen but simply want to look better, feel better, and shed some weight. Even if the motivation for wanting to make a change differs from person to person, everyone has one simple request: *help me burn more fat.*

On the surface, there's nothing wrong with this goal. Fat burning is one way to transform your body, but it's not the only way to shift the numbers on the scale. In fact, burning fat is only half of the equation. The amount of body fat you have is the by-product of two equally important variables—*fat burning* and *fat storage.*

Most diets discuss only fat burning, which gives you a narrow view of your options, and leaves you with a short-sighted, and likely unsustainable and unsatisfying, plan. A diet that limits fat *storage* leads to long-term leanness and health. When it comes to effective dieting, this subtle shift in understanding how to store less fat might be the single most impactful thing you can do. Focusing on minimizing fat storage, and stopping obsessing over fat burning, can lead to dramatic changes for your mind and body.

You might be surprised to hear that minimizing fat storage starts with carbs. Yes, carbs—the villain of diets from keto to Atkins, paleo to Whole30. When it comes to weight loss, carbs are your new heroes.

STOP STORING FAT—BY EATING CARBS!

No matter what your food sources, weight loss and gain are controlled by calorie balance. If you burn more calories than you eat, you will not gain weight. This concept often gets translated into the idea of "move more, eat less." Unfortunately, it's not that simple. The real challenge, as mentioned previously, is about getting away from extremes and misleading outcomes.

When fat burning is greater than fat storage, you lose weight. And, if fat storage is greater than fat burning, you gain weight. It comes down to this question: Is it easier to burn fat or store less fat? Frankly, fat burning requires more time and effort and forces you to cut popular foods out of your diet. It is easier to focus on eating in a way that leads to less fat storage. And in the game of health, a winning strategy is the one that's easier to follow and maintain.

We've all heard that cutting carbs is your best bet if you want to lose weight. And there is some truth to that approach because it can work. But honestly, most people don't enjoy going carb-free and can't keep it up indefinitely. That probably has something to do with pasta, tacos, and pancakes all being so delicious.

When people talk about cutting carbs and saying they lost weight, one or more of the following things is likely the reason: First, most of the weight is water weight loss. Carbs are a sponge for water, so while there may be initial weight loss, it is transient, and the weight inevitably comes back. The second, and perhaps the most impactful for body-fat loss, is the significant increase in calories coming from overeating certain types of carbs. I want you to understand that it's not the overconsumption of quinoa and apples that is leading to weight gain; it's foods like donuts, muffins, and pizza that are the culprits—and on closer examination these foods often have copious amounts of fat. For example, 50 percent of the calories in a donut are from fat and more than 50 percent of the calories in a Pizza Hut pepperoni deep-dish pizza are from fat. These foods are not carbs; rather they are fat-loaded foods that also contain carbohydrates. So if you skip your slice of pizza and lose weight, you are not really losing weight because of cutting carbs, you are losing because of cutting fat.

> No one ever talks about how carbs make it less likely that you *store* fat. That may sound counterintuitive, but the truth—which is backed up by dozens of studies—is that carbs *don't make you fat.*

The bigger problem is that you've been taught that carbs make you fat. But no one ever talks about how carbs make it less likely that you *store* fat. That may sound counterintuitive, but the truth—which is backed up by dozens of studies—is that carbs *don't make you fat.*

When you need energy, your body wants carbs. Now, if your energy tank is full and you take on more food/fuel (think of putting gas into a car), your body must do something with those excess calories. Conventional wisdom says that excess carbs become fat. But your body does not prefer to store carbs as fat. Research shows that when you overeat, approximately 2 percent of the fat stored in your adipose tissue (your fat cells) is from carbohydrates. That means the other 98 percent of fat stored in your body is from *dietary fat.* A high-fat diet (when carbs are low) can help burn more fat—that's the logic behind keto diets. But dietary fat is also your body's preferred form of energy to *store fat.* Meaning, when you eat more fat, your body easily stores more fat. Therefore, although high-fat diets can burn more fat, they also lead to more fat storage. This is something you rarely hear about when people talk about the "benefits" of eliminating carbs from your diet and adding more fats.

I know carbs are blamed for just about everything, but as I've seen with my clients and through my extensive experience, cutting carbs completely is a case of throwing out the baby with the bathwater. Except for sugar, most carbs aren't the problem (we'll get to sugar in chapter 7). But eating less of *one* carb—sugar—does not mean you should abandon *all* carbs. In fact, all carbs are not created equal, and by choosing the right carbs, you will greatly benefit your diet and your waistline.

START BURNING FAT—BY EATING CARBS!

New breakthroughs are often built on the foundations of long-standing, boring science, not one stand-alone new study. And that old science, the stuff everyone likes to ignore, offers a clear picture of what your body needs to function its best, feel amazing, and burn fat.

I first learned that "fat burns in a carbohydrate flame" when I was an undergrad studying nutrition at the University of Western Ontario. The idea came from biochemistry experiments that occurred at the turn of the twentieth century—the 1890s to be exact—when scientists were beginning to understand the basic functioning of our metabolism. The phrase refers to the actual process of burning body fat and the nutrients your body needs to support that process.

While we've made a lot of amazing nutrition discoveries since then, and we now understand so much more about human metabolism and how we can optimize our health, *how* the human body works hasn't changed. The structures identified more than 125 years ago are the same structures that support us today. What was true then is true now: carbohydrates are the fuel that allows your fat-burning machinery to work.

Think of it this way: your body is built to burn energy. Every bit of food you consume is designed to be used intelligently. Protein is composed of chains of amino acids, which do everything from helping you build stronger muscles to supplying the building blocks you need for beautiful hair, skin, and nails. Fats are broken down into fatty acids, which support the proper functioning of your cells, allow chemical signals to transfer effectively, support your brain health, and help balance hormone levels. And carbohydrates—yes, those "terrible" carbs—are the preferred energy source of your body. Your brain, heart, muscles, and digestive system thrive on carbs.

Your body is pretty efficient at burning fat, no matter what your previous dieting experiences might have caused you to believe. However, remember that to burn fat molecules, your body needs glucose. And glucose is provided by you guessed it—carbohydrates. So, while low-carb diets can help increase fat burning (because you're using fat as energy), carbohydrates themselves are the fuel for the fat-burning mechanism in your body.

In one controlled lab study, where participants were kept in a metabolic ward for two weeks to see the impact of a low-carb versus a low-fat diet, the low-fat (higher-carb) group burned more fat. And in a review of thirty-two other fat-loss studies, researchers found the same thing: low-fat, higher-carb diets were more effective for fat loss than low-carb, higher-fat diets. You don't hear much about this, but it paints a clear picture of how we've all been made to believe that carbs are the enemy.

Your brain, heart, muscles, and digestive system thrive on carbs. If your organs and muscles are your engines, carbs are the fuel.

THE POWER OF PASTA AND OTHER CARBS

For many people, the mere thought of pasta elicits a mix of guilt and pleasure. Because pasta is delicious, we assume it can't be good for us. However, if you look at the typical nutrition profile of pasta, nothing jumps out as being problematic. It's moderate in calories, not loaded with sugar, is relatively low in fat, has protein, and is often a decent source of fiber. When I look at pasta, I see all the makings of a balanced, nutrient-filled meal. When most people look at pasta, they see only *carbs*. And because carbs are "bad," then pasta must be fattening and is another food to keep off your plate.

If I can convince you that pasta, as a representative of carbs, is good for you, you're more likely to achieve the mindset shift accomplished by the healthiest people in the world.

The idea that pasta is healthy might be hard to accept . . . until you understand that the science of fat loss and gain starts with how we digest carbs.

EATING PASTA . . . A LITTLE DIGESTION 101

Most pastas, especially whole wheat or multigrain versions—but even traditional versions of spaghetti or fettuccine—mix carbs, protein, fiber, and a little fat. This balance makes all the difference because it affects digestion and how your body absorbs the food.

As you take each bite of fettuccine, spaghetti, or rigatoni you begin the process of fueling your body in ways the low-carb diet industry desperately wants to hide. The function of digestion is as old as time and just as central to your general health as breathing and sleeping. The moment you start eating pasta, I encourage you to enjoy the flavors in your mouth. It's not only important that you appreciate what you are eating but, the more time you spend chewing, the more you unlock the magic of how eating the right foods the right way can keep you full and fuel your body.

The more you chew your food, the more likely you will be satisfied because it slows down your pace (it takes time for the signals in your stomach to tell your brain you're full, which is why fast eaters tend to overeat) and starts a chemical process that is essential to how your digestive system works. As you chew, you create saliva, which has enzymes that break down the molecules that hold the pasta together. The more you chew and enjoy the food, the more the enzymes will prepare the food for a healthier journey.

As the enzymes work their magic, the pasta transforms from the noodles you saw on your plate into a mixture of different sugars and a wide variety of other nutrients, including fiber, vitamins, and minerals. If you've mixed your pasta with some olive oil and protein—as I recommend you do—you're preparing your digestive system to use what your body needs and remove what it doesn't.

Once the enzymes do their job, the pasta is on its way to support your body. Because of the combination of fiber, vitamins, protein, and fat, the good news is that the nutrients are in no hurry to hit your stomach. The more slowly food moves to your stomach, the more you will feel satisfied. That's how you stay full and curb hunger and cravings, which is part of the power of pasta (and other carbs). This puts you in a prime position to *use* your food rather than store it.

You don't need all the details, but by the time the pasta hits your stomach, your body shuttles different types of sugar—from glucose to fructose—to help fuel your body. These sugars can cause a slight increase in blood sugar, but don't worry; this is completely normal. It happens when you eat almost anything.

Consuming pasta might also cause a slight increase in insulin. Excess insulin production can surely be detrimental for some people, but a small spike—the kind you get from eating pasta—is completely normal; insulin is a necessary hormone in your body. You *need* insulin largely because it helps with using and storing energy. Without insulin, the broken-down sugars would sit in your bloodstream making you hyperglycemic (chronic high blood sugar), which can cause organ problems and other damage to your body. But, when insulin works as it should, the sugars are transported to the cells, where your body needs them most—to fuel your mind, body, or muscles.

That's your body on pasta—efficiently using the nutrients in your meal to give the energy your organs and body systems need to function. That's why research suggests that regular pasta eaters tend to be healthier. In an analysis of the diets of more than eighty thousand women, scientists found that women with higher pasta consumption (an average of three times per week) had a lower incidence of heart disease and stroke.[6]

Now, this doesn't mean that eating pasta prevents disease or keeps you lean. But it does mean that you can eat pasta regularly, without guilt, and still be healthy, fit, and able to fight off disease.

BREAKING BREAD

Bread has a terrible reputation. But much like pasta, that bad rep is mostly unearned. If you dig into research about bread, you will quickly discover that it has no negative impact on overall health, or that the impact is overwhelmingly positive. In fact, if you look at multigrains, whole wheat, sourdough, and other variations of bread, you discover that eating bread is associated with a lower incidence of type 2 diabetes, cardiovascular disease, and cancer.

One study suggests that eating the equivalent of 7½ slices of whole grain bread per day is associated with optimal health.[7] Bread is an integral piece of the Mediterranean diet, which has incredible health outcomes.[8] In other words, it's time to appreciate bread as another healthy carb that you can include in your diet. If you need help finding the best ones, Harvard researchers suggest approximately 2 grams of fiber for every 15 grams of carbohydrates in the bread you select.[9]

Here are some tasty and healthy breads:

- Ezekiel bread
- Pumpernickel bread
- Rye bread
- 100% whole grain whole wheat bread
- Buckwheat bread
- Spelt bread
- Sourdough bread
- Soda bread
- Flaxseed bread
- Porridge oat bread[10]

Of course, bread and pasta don't represent your only choices when it comes to carbs: quality carbs come in all shapes and sizes and are some of the healthiest things you can eat. (See a full list of options on page 32.)

- Fruits
- Vegetables
- Whole grains
- Legumes
- Tubers (potato family)

The Mediterranean diet, which has a good amount of research supporting its claims to help maintain a healthy weight and reduce the likelihood of heart disease and other cardiovascular diseases, is a diet that features all healthy carb options.[11] Specifically, the ten healthiest countries worldwide all follow a high-carb diet. That doesn't mean they're eating pizza and donuts. They enjoy bread and rice, pasta and grains, beans and lentils, which are linked to improved overall health, longevity, and fat loss.

NOT ALL CARBS ARE CREATED EQUAL

I don't believe in demonizing one food over another, but I do think that there are better choices that you can make over the carbs you are adding to your diet. You'll notice that I said "choices" because I believe that you should be in the driver's seat regarding the foods you put on your plate and the path you take to better health. I really want you to embrace, not abuse, carbs and see them as a significant part of your healthy diet and weight management goals. As you'll see from the discussion of sugar in chapter 7, eating all carbs all the time isn't what we are going for here. Complex carbs like whole grains and vegetables are central to *The Carb Reset* plan. Things like donuts, cakes, and cookies (which also happen to be calorically dense) are not the type of carbs that will sustain you on your journey to good health, but they can be something that you enjoy periodically and will not take you off your path to your health goals. Making the choices makes the difference.

Another food group that has suffered from the paranoia about eating carbs is vegetables. In the next chapter, we'll dig into the reasons why a variety of vegetables are good for you—especially those that are rich in carbs.

CHAPTER 4

All Veggies, All the Time

A = ALL THE VEGGIES

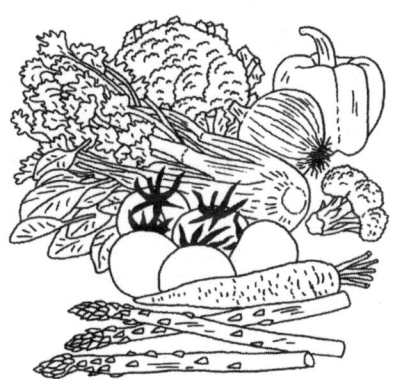

The message of this chapter is simple—eat your vegetables! I know a lot of people struggle with eating vegetables. That's okay! In general, I want you to focus on having vegetables in at least two of your meals each day. And, when you do, feel free to pile them up. If you are not a big fan of vegetables, check out the recipes in chapter 10 for ideas on how to incorporate more of them into your life.

I'm sure you have heard of diets, and possibly been on one, that outright forbid eating certain vegetables like red peppers, sweet potatoes, butternut squashes, peas, or carrots (largely due to that good old fear of their innate sugars, or carbs). *The Carb Reset* does not banish these delicious and healthy vegetables from your plate, but instead makes them a welcome part of your diet. Frankly, no one has ever gotten obese from eating bell peppers or carrots.

WHAT MOM NEVER TOLD YOU: THE BENEFITS OF EATING YOUR VEGETABLES

The great thing about vegetables is that they are high in water, fiber, vitamins, and minerals, and are generally low in calories. High fiber fills you up and can help suppress your appetite. You'll get fuller faster, and that feeling will last longer. And high water content helps you stay hydrated. Vegetables also have low calorie density so you can eat a lot without breaking the calorie bank. And, if that isn't enough, they are packed with micronutrients (that is, vitamins and minerals like potassium and magnesium) that can support your general health as well as promote a healthy metabolism.

WEIGHT LOSS

There is evidence that there is an inverse relationship between vegetable consumption and weight. The more vegetables you eat, the lighter you are! These benefits are found largely through eating higher-fiber vegetables, but even lower-fiber vegetables aren't linked to weight gain. A study found that "phytochemicals in F&V [fruits and vegetables] have been found to act as anti-obesity agents because they may play a role in suppressing growth of adipose tissue." Adipose tissue is body fat. You want less of it, so eat more veggies.[1]

In addition, the compounds, nutrients, and phytonutrients in vegetables and fruits can also help to *burn* fat.

DIGESTION

Eating food with high fiber and water content like vegetables supports your gut health. Fiber is a prebiotic that helps promote the growth of probiotics, which are the helpful bacteria in your gut and digestive tract. Probiotics are beneficial microbes that maintain health and can reduce the number of harmful microbes (germs) in your digestive system. They can also contribute to maintaining a healthy microbiome. A study from the Mayo Clinic found that "a healthy gut microbiome helps with digestion, boosts the immune system, contributes to blood sugar levels, and may even influence mood and mental health."[2]

An increased intake of dietary fiber is also beneficial because it reduces the length of time that food remains in your digestive tract. Basically, it helps to move things along, keeping you regular. In addition to helping to reduce bloated or crampy feelings from constipation, this is good because fecal matter that stays too long in your tract can ferment and has been associated with digestive cancers.

Indeed, vegetables—particularly those that are green, red, purple, or white—can help in the prevention of colon cancer. Fruit, because it is high in fiber and water, is also linked to a reduction in colon cancer risks.

HOW MUCH SHOULD YOU EAT?

A study from the Harvard Medical School found that five servings of vegetables a day lowered the risk of death, heart disease or stroke, cancer, and respiratory disease. Eating more fruits and vegetables beyond that didn't provide any additional benefit in lowering the risk of death.[3] However, because it's very difficult to overeat vegetables, eating fruits and vegetables beyond the recommended five servings a day might have additional weight management benefits due to their relatively low caloric density and high satiety quotient (they fill you up!).

Another plus about vegetables is that they don't have to be exotic or hard to find for them to have benefits to your health. Whatever vegetable is readily available in your local grocer's produce aisle or farmers' market is a vegetable you should eat to your heart's content. Even canned and frozen vegetables can be a healthier choice than no veggies at all.

To be clear, I'm not talking about eating vegetables that are smothered in high-fat dressings, dips, or sauces. Loading up veggies with these things defeats the beneficial purpose of eating vegetables in the first place—especially if the sauces or dips are loaded with fat (more on fats in the next chapter).

Of course, in the recipe section, I have some pointers on how to best prepare vegetables to maximize their taste and nutritional value. You can eat vegetables raw, steamed, baked, pureed, grilled, sautéed, and even mixed into pasta sauce, smoothies, and more. The many possibilities can help you expand your palate without expanding your waistline.

THE POWER OF LEGUMES

Legumes, a member of the vegetable family, generally include beans, peas, and lentils. They have protein (more on protein in chapter 6), fiber, fat, antioxidants, carbs, and vitamins. Good for heart health and a great option for a plant-based protein, they play an essential role in a healthy diet that is carb-rich. Great beans and legumes include:

Chickpeas (Garbanzo beans)
Navy beans
Lentils
Soybeans (Edamame)
Fava beans
Kidney beans
Black beans
Pinto beans
Cannellini beans

A staple of many diets around the world—including the Mediterranean and many Asian diets (in countries that boast some of the healthiest populations around the globe)—beans are filling, nutritious, relatively inexpensive, easy to prepare, and provide a lot of bang for the buck for adding protein and fiber to a meal.

Nearly 92 percent of U.S. adults do not include legumes as part of their diets. Which is a shame because legumes are not only tasty but high in fiber and contribute to satiety, as well as gut health. They are almost a perfect food in and of themselves and contain a host of micronutrients—carbs, fiber, protein, B vitamins, iron, copper, magnesium, manganese, zinc, and phosphorus. They are virtually free of saturated fat. One serving of legumes (½ cup) contains 115 calories, 20 grams of carbs, 7–9 grams of fiber, 8 grams of protein, and 1 gram of fat—no nutrition bar on the market can come close to that!

According to the American Diabetes Association, "Along with being a highly nutritious food, evidence shows that legumes can play an important role in the prevention and management of a number of health conditions . . . ,"[4] which include lowering total and LDL cholesterol, supporting weight management, and benefiting blood pressure management.

Eating beans can be good for those with type 2 diabetes because legumes can help to increase glycemic and lipid control. In one study, participants consumed a cup of legumes as part of their daily diet and after three months, their A1C (which is a measure of blood sugar levels) significantly decreased, along with lowering their total cholesterol and blood pressure.[5]

A study in *Advances in Nutrition* found, "A higher legume intake was associated with lower mortality from all causes and stroke, but no association was observed for CVD [cardiovascular disease], CHD [coronary heart disease], and cancer mortality. These results support dietary recommendations to increase the consumption of legumes."[6]

Increasing the amount of vegetables and beans you eat daily is a great way to fill you up, get your digestion moving, be heart healthy, promote gut health, and add some essential nutrients and vitamins to your plate.

Next, we'll take a look at fats and how best to use them in *The Carb Reset*, with some specific guidance on avoiding added and saturated fats.

CHAPTER 5

Fat Facts

T = A THUMB OF FAT

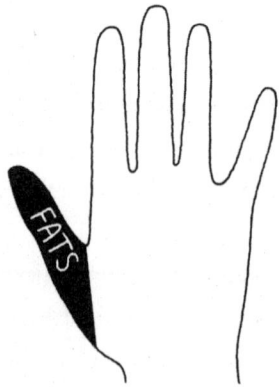

FATS

Let's get one thing clear: fat is essential for our bodies to function, and many quality sources of fat (when consumed in moderation) won't necessarily make you fat.

When they are metabolized, fats break down into fatty acids, which support the proper functioning of your cells, allow chemical signals to transfer effectively, support your brain health, and help with hormone levels. When it comes to calories, however, no macronutrient is as calorie dense as fat. Every gram of fat has more than twice as many calories as a single gram of carbohydrates or protein. Obviously, then, when you eat fats in excess, they can play a big role in adding lots of sneaky calories to your diet. The good news is that you don't need to cut out *all* the fat; you need to cut down on *added* fats (oils) and *saturated* fat.

Using the right, good-quality fats and oils in your diet sets the foundation for positive change. When you eat more of what's healthy, less of what's potentially dangerous, and limit the quantity of fats so you don't trigger your brain to drive you to be an eating machine, you can transform how your brain reacts to food. Instead of getting too many calories from added fats, you have the ideal amount of everything your body needs to feel full and burn body fat without losing your way.

HOW *ADDED* FATS HAVE MADE US FAT

The low-carb/Atkins/keto movement was all about eating more fat. So manufacturers put more fat into everything, and we loaded up our plates in the way my friend at In-N-Out Burger did: double cheese-burger with bacon and no bun. Now, as food scientists move to create more plant-based meats like Beyond Meat and Impossible, they are using vegetable oils to make up the bulk of their calories. In fact, too many foods—especially those that are ultraprocessed—are loaded with fats from *vegetable oils*. That might sound healthy—there is the word *vegetable* in there, after all—but the vegetable oil amounts in highly pro-cessed foods are actually not so healthy at all.

According to USDA data, calorie consumption from the 1970s to 2014 has increased by anywhere from 600 to 700 calories, and the con-sumption of added fats and oils jumped from 53 pounds per year (per person) to more than 86 pounds per year during that same time period. That's *a lot* of added calories.[1]

To give you an idea of what many people in the United States are eating, on the next page is a recent breakdown of the American diet looks like as a percentage of daily calories—note the high percentage of fats and vegetable oils.[2]

Keep in mind that with beef, lamb, veal, poultry, and dairy (butter) more than half the calories in these foods come from fat—unless you are eating lean cuts of meat.

That breakdown doesn't look terrible. That is, until you compare the intake of *added fats* with the surge in obesity in the United States. Unfortunately, our added fat intake has been on a steady increase since

Nutrients and Their Percentage of Daily Calories in the Average American Diet

Wheat, corn, rice, and grains: 23%

Fat/vegetable oils: 21%

Added sugar: 15%

Dairy: 9%

Beef, lamb, veal: 6%

Poultry: 5%

Pork: 4%

Potatoes: 3%

Fruits: 3%

Vegetables: 2%

Nuts: 2%

Eggs: 2%

Animal fats: 2% (butter)

Fruit juice: 1%

Fish: 1%

the 1980s, and the correlation with obesity rates has as well. My approach to eating the right fats—along with carbs, veggies, and proteins—will help you to avoid or to reverse this trend and get on a better path to health.

Added fats parallel the U.S. obesity and diabetes epidemic better than a correlation with overall macronutrients or sugar. The amount of added fat has increased by 28 percent, whereas carbs and sugar have decreased since 1999. When you put it all together, the increase in weight gain is a factor of too much added fat and too much added sugar in diets that are low in protein, carbs, and fiber. To make matters worse, foods that combine high added fats (think oils) and high added sugars rewire your brain to desire that type of food, so you keep eating . . . and eating . . . and eating.

If that wasn't enough, eating like this makes it easier to consume too much saturated fat. As with most things, while some saturated fat is okay, too much is not. A twenty-five-year study of more than twelve thousand people found that diets higher in saturated fat are linked to heart disease mortality, cardiovascular problems, high LDL cholesterol, and high blood pressure.[3] Replacing dietary fat—and saturated fat, in particular—with healthier carb sources can have a life-changing impact. In fact, in one study of more than a hundred thousand people, simply replacing 5 percent of calories from saturated fat with whole grain carbohydrates led to a 25 percent decrease in heart disease risk.[4]

CHOOSING HEALTHY FATS

When I tell clients that they need to include healthier fats in their diets, they immediately question what the definition of *healthier* is. Should I load up on nuts? What about coconut oil? Olive oil? Butter?

To understand the "healthy fat" debate, you need to hit refresh on the extremes ("Fat is bad!" or "Fat is amazing!") and take a different perspective. Not only will this new approach give you peace of mind but it will also help you understand what you can eat often, what is okay in moderate doses, and what you should completely avoid.

First, let's get clear on what we're talking about when we're talking about fats. There are three kinds, and I'm putting them here in the order they should be in your diet:

Unsaturated fats—found in nuts, seeds, and vegetable oils. The good fat! Within reason (as you'll see in my recipes), you should not be afraid of this kind of fat.

Saturated fats—found in beef, pork, chicken, coconut and palm oils. You need these fats in certain quantities.

Trans fats—found in fried and ultraprocessed foods like French fries, cookies, and cakes. Can you eat a cookie a day like me? Of course! But if you change one thing about your diet, start here. These are the kinds of fats that have very little redeeming value.

Just a reminder that calling something "healthy" is relative—what may be good for you may not be good for someone else, and this may largely be a function of genetics and lifestyle. But I'm encouraging you to make eating choices that are based on the best information that we have and that lead to recommendations for what is healthy for most people. There's also plenty of research to help you figure that out.

A study called the PREDIMED, which followed thousands of people over several years, showed that olive oil and nuts were linked with better overall cardiovascular health.[5] By definition, both would be considered healthy fats. The same is true for avocados (and avocado oil), fish, and nut butters. All these foods contain beneficial health properties over and above their fat content. These are the fat sources you want to eat most often.

You can add some variety, but certain fats shouldn't be consumed in large amounts. A perfect example is coconut oil, which seemed to explode in popularity after a study suggested that coconut oil might inhibit the growth of certain problematic bacteria.[6] Next thing you know, people were rubbing coconut oil in their hair and all over their bodies.

Most of the hype over healthy fats concerns a compound known as MCT, aka medium-chain triglyceride, which people tout as a fat burner because of the way the fat is broken down in your body. MCTs are found in coconut oil (you can isolate them), but they are not the same thing as coconut oil. MCTs can have health benefits, but their reputation for melting fat from your body is significantly overstated.

One study showed that men who ate more MCTs lost a whopping one-quarter of a pound per month more than those who followed a "regular" diet each month.[7] Suddenly, there was a trend of adding coconut oil to everything from coffee creamers to salad dressings. But here's the thing. Burning one more pound of fat every four months does not mean you are experiencing a fat-loss miracle. And yet, that was the takeaway.

If that wasn't enough to make you suspicious of these purported benefits, when a different group of researchers examined whether coconut oil had the same effect as MCT, they found that they could not replicate the study.[8]

Coconut oil's glowing reputation is so unearned that in 2017, the American Heart Association (AHA) released a report advising against the consistent consumption of it.[9] The biggest concern cited in the AHA report is that coconut oil is high in saturated fat. But anyone who has even casually glanced at a coconut oil nutrition facts label would know that—it's stated right on the label. And while saturated fat has been blamed wrongly for a lot of health problems, it's also not something you should eat in limitless amounts.[10] Instead, as I say above, you'll want the majority of your fats to come from unsaturated sources and the minority from saturated fats.

Additionally, a review of fourteen different studies on MCT oil found that in eight of the studies there was no weight loss whatsoever, and in four of the studies participants burned a few extra calories but scale weight didn't change.[11] If you want to burn money (MCT isn't cheap) to lose an extra pound, you can. But there are better ways to do so.

Conversely, canola oil deserves a mention here because of its undeserved bad reputation. Many people fear using canola oil over concerns about consuming too many omega-6 fatty acids. It turns out, however, that omega-6 fatty acids can be good for your health. Research in forty-two studies found that canola oil led to a significant improvement in multiple blood lipid (fat) markers, including a reduction in total cholesterol, LDL cholesterol, and several other markers compared with all other oils.[12] Much of the concern regarding the omega-6 fatty acids found in canola oil is based on animal research, but human trials suggest omega-6s don't increase inflammation in people as they do in animals.[13]

More important, the real issue—as we've discussed—is that oils are easy to overeat, are energy dense (loaded with many calories), and tend to be found in many ultraprocessed foods that lack nutritional benefits. So if you eat *a lot* of oils, you can expect bad health outcomes because you're eating many foods that aren't great for your health—but that doesn't mean a particular amount of canola is bad for you.

If you choose to cook with canola oil, just know that it's very low in saturated fat, high in monounsaturated fat, and has phytosterols, which help limit the absorption of cholesterol in your body. If you prefer cooking with other oils—such as olive or avocado—that's a great decision, too.

Remember, no single food is going to make or break your diet. You've been taught to view foods as "good" or "bad," but that's a gross oversimplification. Much like sugar, fat in your diet is about understanding what you should eat often and what you should eat infrequently.

HOW TO MAKE FAT WORK FOR YOU

When you use the PATH approach to put food on your plate, it helps to follow a few simple rules. First and foremost, you want to make sure you include fat in your diet and—per the acronym—a thumb-size portion at every meal, which amounts to about a tablespoon of fat or oil, for example, as part of a salad dressing or cooking oil, combined.

The healthiest fats to eat in great quantities are olive oil, nuts, avocados, fatty fish (like salmon), and seeds. These contain polyunsaturated and monounsaturated fats, which have health benefits that have been supported by many studies.

You should know that you can't game the system by simply adding a "healthy" fat source to an otherwise bad diet (one that's high in calorie-dense packaged foods and low in fruits, vegetables, and whole foods). In fact, it could make you less healthy if the additional calories you pile onto that unhealthy diet take you over your daily caloric intake. Too much fat and oil are where calories sneak in and can lead to weight gain. In my PATH plan, fat will be a part of your diet, but you'll be eating it throughout the day, and not in large quantities.

When you use oil in cooking, it's better to use unsaturated fat, such as olive oil. It's also best to buy the extra virgin version of any oil. Doing so will ensure you're buying a quality oil that will work well for your body.

If you're going to use saturated fats—like coconut oil or butter—

you can use them in moderation, but they shouldn't be your primary source of fat or be used in all your cooking. A word (or two) on saturated fat: historically, a connection has been made between saturated fats and heart disease, but there is more recent research that suggests that saturated fat is not to blame for cardiovascular diseases.[14] It is possible that there is a correlation effect in that by eating more calorically dense foods—those high in saturated fat—instead of high-water, high-fiber, nutrient-dense foods, there may be health consequences. What do these contradictory findings mean for you? Because I advocate moderation, when it comes to saturated fat, consume it sparingly, as you would any other fat.

Protein plays a role in *The Carb Reset*, but rather than being the central aspect of your diet (as it is with some extreme diets), in the next chapter I'll show how protein will work with other nutrients, especially carbs, to allow you to create a balanced plate.

CHAPTER 6

Protein Power

H = HAND OF PROTEIN

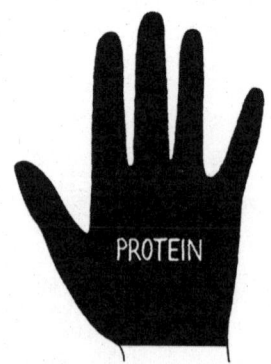

PROTEIN

Although it may seem as if I have a beef (ha!) with eating a mega-high-protein diet, the truth is I advocate for a relatively high-protein diet but promote leaner sources of protein in lieu of their fatty cousins. There is no doubt that protein plays a significant role in your overall health as well as gives support to your weight-loss goals. However, eating only protein to the exclusion of other major nutrients like carbs and healthy fats will not get you where you want to go. Don't get me wrong, protein is good for you, but the best benefits come when it is eaten in combination with other foods.

Proteins are made from chains of amino acids. Our bodies can make only certain kinds of amino acids on their own—these are called nonessential amino acids, and there are eleven kinds of them. Another nine amino acids are considered "essential," but can come only from food sources. The foods that contain the essential amino acids are known as *complete proteins* and include poultry, beef, fish, dairy, eggs, buckwheat, quinoa, and soy.

Protein packs a powerful punch to support your health in so many ways:

- It helps develop stronger muscles (it's nearly impossible to transform the composition of your body, build muscle, and become stronger without protein in your diet).
- It is essential for cell repair (and can aid in injury recovery).
- It supports bone health (both during bone growth and to maintain bone mass, which reduces the risk for osteoporosis).
- It fosters organ growth (and maintains organs' healthy functioning).
- It helps to maintain the immune system (it makes antibodies that can fight off infection).
- It is a nutrient that helps your body make red blood cells.
- It plays a part in regulating hormones (growth, energy, appetite).
- It supplies the vital nutrients you need for healthy hair, skin, and nails.

HIGH-PROTEIN DIETS AND WEIGHT LOSS

As if all those benefits weren't enough, consuming adequate protein in the diet is associated with weight loss. An article in the *Journal of Obesity & Metabolic Syndrome* noted that "several clinical trials have found that consuming more protein than the recommended dietary allowance not only reduces body weight (BW) . . . [but] HPD [high-protein diet] is an effective and safe tool for weight reduction that can prevent obesity and obesity-related diseases."[1]

One of the ways that protein works this magic is that it can help you to feel full as well as less hungry. It does this by reducing the hormone ghrelin, which regulates hunger, and increasing the hormones that make you feel full. Consuming protein can also have lasting effects on your desire to eat—one study of overweight men showed that by increasing protein in their diets, they experienced fewer cravings and had a decreased desire for nighttime snacking.[2] Because protein helps you feel full, eating it effectively controls snacking, which can contribute to eating fewer calories throughout the day. And, of course, consuming fewer calories can ultimately lead to weight loss.

Additionally, a diet with a high level of protein can induce thermogenesis, which increases energy expenditure. During thermogenesis, your body burns calories as it digests proteins. It does not take as much energy to digest other foods, so you are essentially boosting your metabolism and burning more calories when you eat protein than you do when you eat other foods.[3]

If you want to build muscle mass and improve strength, protein is crucial—especially if you want to build up strength while also losing weight. If you cut down on protein while trying to lose weight, you run the risk of losing muscle mass at the same time. Maintaining muscles can also contribute to a boost in your metabolism so you will burn more calories at rest than someone with less muscle mass. Furthermore, having adequate protein in your diet can help prevent potential muscle loss that can occur as you grow older. So diets high in protein can help you reduce body weight and enhance body composition. And, once you have lost weight, a diet that has protein can also help you keep that weight off over time.

Over the years, I've worked with many female clients who have been very gun-shy about adding more protein to their diets. They have been led to believe that protein is for people who are trying to create bulk and build big bodies. They've seen and heard about protein powders and weight-gaining supplements that are marketed to build big muscles and conclude that protein has no place on their plates. I always try to reassure these clients that this fear of protein is not founded in science and, in fact, consuming protein might actually be critical to their reaching their weight-loss goals and maintaining them.

Diets high in protein can help you reduce body weight and enhance body composition. And, once you have lost weight, a diet that has protein can also help you keep that weight off over time.

One memorable client had been a vegan most of her life, and although she had plenty of plant-based choices for putting protein on her plate (see below), let's just say she wasn't taking advantage of them. In reality, she ate very little protein at all. The result was that she was exhausted, had skin issues, her hair was falling out, and she struggled with her body composition. And although she was small in stature, she had a relatively high body-fat percentage.

As we worked together, she agreed to increase her dietary protein intake, and in the process, she started to feel a lot better. Not only that, she also started looking the way she wanted to look. The protein didn't bulk up her muscles, but it helped her to have more energy and added to an overall improvement in her health.

SOURCES OF PROTEIN

The *H* in the acronym PATH stands for a "hand" of protein. But not all sources of protein are equal. If meat or poultry appeals to you, always choose lean cuts of these options. Red meat, in particular, can be high in fat, which can be detrimental to cardiovascular health and weight loss. There is also a strong link between red meat consumption and various forms of cancer.[4]

I also recommend that you steer clear of eating too many processed meats like bacon, hot dogs, salamis, or deli meats—largely because they can have a high salt content and be loaded with preservatives. Too much sodium has been associated with stroke, high blood pressure, and heart disease.[5]

Seafood is one of my favorite sources of dietary protein. Shellfish such as lobster, shrimp, and crab are among the leanest sources of dietary protein available. Other seafood such as salmon, sardines, and mackerel are loaded with quality protein and healthy omega-3 fatty acids. Fish also provides benefits to the brain, heart, bones, and skin.[6]

Many people choose not to eat meat (animal protein) for a wide range of reasons (environmental, philosophical, religious, for example). If you have chosen not to include animal-based products in your diet, protein can and should still be a part of your dietary plan. If you follow a vegetarian or vegan diet, you can eat plant proteins (like soy and grains) and get the benefits that protein offers your body. But if you are getting your protein from plant-based sources, be sure to eat a variety of those foods, because while meat-based protein is a complete protein, most plant-based sources of protein do not have all the amino acids your body requires. They do, however, often have the added benefit of fiber, which can help you to feel full.

PLANT-BASED SOURCES OF PROTEIN

Plant-based sources of protein include vegetables like legumes, and whole grains, which are not only great sources of protein but also provide health-promoting fiber, vitamins, and minerals. While most vegetarian sources of protein are low in fat, including saturated fat, I urge you to beware of added coconut fat or vegan versions of animal proteins such as veggie burgers. These are often loaded with additional oils, so check the labels.

There are many choices of meat replacements that look, feel, and taste like meat, although they are made from plant sources. If you miss the taste of meat, these are not bad options, but be aware that while meatless burgers are a good source of protein, minerals, and vitamins, they are also heavily processed and are high in saturated fat.[7] Also note that plant-based milks, especially oat milk, receive most of their calories from added vegetable oil.

So if you are a carnivore, omnivore, or herbivore, you can find sources of protein that will support your health and round out your diet. (In chapter 10, I will provide a list of vegetarian swaps so you can find protein-rich foods that suit your lifestyle.)

GREAT SOURCES OF PROTEIN

MEAT: lean beef

POULTRY: lean chicken, lean turkey (skinless)

SEAFOOD: salmon, shrimp, trout, scallops, octopus

DAIRY: low-fat/nonfat milk, Greek/Icelandic yogurt, kefir, cottage cheese

EGGS AND EGG WHITES

LEGUMES: chickpeas, lentils (also high in fiber)

SOY: tofu, edamame, tempeh, soy milk

GRAINS: quinoa, millet, teff, sorghum, spelt, kamut, whole wheat

NUTS AND NUT BUTTERS

VEGETABLES: broccoli, spinach, peas, seaweed, zucchini, cucumbers[8, 9, 10]

While some diets may promote eating primarily protein—think of my friend and his double cheeseburger with bacon (no bun)—protein works best in balance with other nutrients like carbs, vegetables, and a little bit of healthy fat.

Next, we'll examine how sugar (in moderation) can be a part of your healthy diet.

CHAPTER 7

The Scoop on Sugar

Although sugar is not specifically part of the PATH approach to filling your plate, I mention it because I get asked about it all the time—largely because sugar gets a lot of bad press; many people think they need to avoid it altogether. The reality is that your body is designed to need and use some sugar (key word *some*) because it is a valuable energy source that fuels your brain and muscles and helps the process of burning fat. When you eat carbohydrates (any carbohydrates, vegetables included), your body eventually breaks them down into glucose (aka sugar), which the body uses as fuel. If you don't have any sugar in your diet, your body manufactures it (even if you avoid all carbohydrates) by converting dietary protein and body fat, or stealing from your muscle tissue. So the idea that *all* sugar is bad when your body is designed to use it and convert it into energy doesn't make sense.

The problem isn't sugar itself, but *too much sugar* and *added sugar*. Knowing which sugars you need to limit and which ones have a place in your diet will allow you to add more diversity and happiness to what you eat, and will also help you stress less about every gram of sugar you eat. In fact, science doesn't support the idea that you need to avoid all sugar, all the time.

But, judging from what I hear from clients, nothing seems to give people more guilt than sugar. Anytime they enjoy something sweet with sugar—even if it's for a great reason, like having a slice of birthday cake—they beat themselves up, feel like they've broken their diet, and put themselves at risk for developing a poor relationship with food.

They have bought into the idea that sugar is "toxic" and consuming it, in any form, is like ingesting poison. Calling sugar toxic can get attention-grabbing headlines, but it doesn't make it true. The fact is that sugar's actual "toxicity" level is approximately six pounds per day. I really enjoy my daily chocolate chip cookie, but not even the biggest sweet tooth could consume six pounds of sugar each day. Another aspect of sugar's alleged toxicity is its addictive nature. The anti-sugar crowd likes to compare it with addictive drugs. If you were to eat a spoonful of sugar (cue Mary Poppins), how much would you want to shovel down a second, third, or fourth spoonful? The answer is that most people wouldn't, because sugar alone isn't particularly palatable. Additionally, sugar is not inherently fattening. A gram of sugar is 4 calories. And 4 calories, all on their own, will not make you fat.

What's the problem then? Sugar becomes a problem when it's added to foods where it doesn't belong, especially those with a lot of fat and salt.[1] When sugar is combined with other ingredients, it creates the sweet spot—no pun intended—that causes you to become hungrier and triggers a desire to eat even more sugar. Again, it's not the sugar but the high-fat foods (sweet and savory alike) that become problematic. These foods combine sweet, starch, and fat to create confections (or concoctions) that feel good in your mouth, have a pleasing texture, and often have a lot of salt (which helps everything taste better).

Foods that are artificially loaded with sugar are all too easy to overconsume. In fact, you can consume a lot of sugar when it's combined with fat and salt and still not feel full. The typical pattern goes something like this: you eat some sugar (usually combined with other ingredients and hidden in beverages), and then eat some more, and then some more, and next thing you know a box of cookies, a couple cans of soda, and a sugary coffee drink are all gone . . . and you still feel hungry. There is no satiety with added sugar—it doesn't fill you up.

Avoiding processed foods with *added* sugar is central to reducing your sugar intake and bringing more balance to your diet. It is not, as many diets would lead you to believe, avoiding eating fruits and vegetables.

In general, research suggests you can enjoy anywhere from 6 to 12 teaspoons of *added* sugar per day (but it's probably better to have fewer). Just for some perspective: a yogurt loaded with added sugar can take up more than half of your daily allowance of sugar, and one can of regular soda or a 10-ounce glass of orange juice is the equivalent of your *entire daily recommendation* for added sugar. Your body doesn't want or need lots of *added* sugar being poured into everything from granola to pasta sauce, and every food in between.

Sucrose (aka white table sugar, which is 50 percent fructose and 50 percent glucose) and the much-vilified high-fructose corn syrup (which is typically 55 percent fructose and 45 percent glucose) are pretty easy to spot on ingredient labels. But keep in mind that added sugar is sugar no matter how healthy or natural its form may seem. Don't be fooled into thinking honey or maple syrup or agave are better for you than plain old white table sugar. Especially treacherous are sugars in liquid form—sodas, bottled ice teas, and so on. You can drink and drink and drink mass quantities of them—enough calories to account for a five-course meal—and still feel hungry.[2] Perhaps it's unsurprising that soft drinks are linked to the current obesity epidemic.[3] Soda, energy, and sports drinks are by far the main source of added sugar in the average American's diet, accounting for 34.4 percent of the added sugar consumed by adults and children in the United States. Fruit juices aren't any healthier. In fact, they can be even worse because the sugar in fruit juice is fructose, which can stress the liver (only the liver can metabolize fructose in large amounts). While milk contains sugar (lactose, a disaccharide of glucose and galactose), it has far less sugar than fruit juice. Moreover, milk also contains two different proteins and fat, which increase satiety and therefore make it much more difficult to drink excessive amounts of milk versus sweet fruit juice.

Avoiding processed foods with *added* sugar is central to reducing your sugar intake and bringing more balance to your diet. It is not, as many diets would lead you to believe, avoiding eating fruits and vegetables.

CARBS, SUGAR, AND INSULIN

We can't really talk about carbs and sugar without talking about insulin. Insulin is a hormone secreted by the pancreas and released into the bloodstream when glucose levels go up, as happens after eating. It helps glucose get to the cells of the body, where it can be used for energy or stored for future use. Insulin also helps regulate sugar in the bloodstream. When you ingest too much sugar (especially added sugars), you'll have a spike in insulin production as well. Too much of this combination can cause damage to your body. Hyperglycemia (high blood sugar) can cause cell damage, heart issues, strokes, and kidney damage, and chronic high blood sugar can lead to developing type 2 diabetes. Of course, it's bad to have too little as well; low blood sugar can cause dizziness, mental fog, hunger, and weakness.

There's a popular scientific theory—the carbohydrate-insulin model (CIM)—that suggests we get fat because of insulin and not because of too many calories. This theory leads to people stressing about blood sugar, wearing glucose monitors, and freaking out every time their insulin levels fluctuate the slightest bit. Insulin fluctuations are a normal physiological response to when you eat a meal. It's only an issue if insulin stays elevated. Insulin is affected by the foods you eat—protein and fiber will slow the increase in insulin that can occur from eating carbohydrate-containing foods (which is why fiber, found in carbohydrates, is great to include in your diet). Insulin inhibits fat oxidation (fat burning), but that doesn't mean it leads to fat storage. Lots of research shows that higher-carb diets that increase insulin still result in weight loss.

HOW TO REDUCE *ADDED* SUGAR

As I hope is clear by now, you don't need to remove all sugar from your diet; you need to limit *added* sugar. If you can cut down on extra sugar, you will be less likely to feel addicted to super tasty sweets and treats, you'll consume considerably fewer calories, and you'll drop pounds easily. To successfully reduce your sugar habit, don't stress cutting out every gram of sugar. Instead, become more aware of where high amounts of added sugar are hiding in the foods you eat. If you cut out sugar from traditionally savory foods, then you will have room in your diet to truly enjoy sweets. Just like me and my chocolate chip cookie.

Following is a list of foods that are notoriously and surprisingly high in added sugar. There may be some shocks on this list, and some may be your favorite foods. Because *The Carb Reset* is all about flexibility, you don't have to eliminate them from your diet, especially if you love them. But you can reduce their use or seek out versions with less added sugar.

- Flavored yogurt
- Pasta sauce
- Ketchup
- Sweetened cereal
- Breakfast bar
- Barbecue sauce
- Fruit juice and green juice
- Flavored coffee
- Canned soup
- Flavored oatmeal
- Trail mix
- Salad dressing

WHAT ABOUT ARTIFICIAL SWEETENERS?

Artificial sweeteners have been demonized by many, but research has shown they are not as bad as we've been led to believe. Most of the negative research about diet sodas is conducted with rats. But, when humans are tested, the negative results are not replicated. However, if research doesn't support the idea that diet soda causes weight gain directly (seriously, diet soda does not make you fat), plenty of people still believe it disrupts insulin sensitivity and, thereby, makes it easier to store fat.

In a recent study, participants had two drinks per day of either an artificially sweetened drink or carbonated water. The artificially sweetened drink contained aspartame and acesulfame K (what you'd find in your favorite diet beverage, regardless of whether you're a Diet Coke or Diet Pepsi fan). Guess what? After twelve weeks, there was no difference in insulin sensitivity, body weight, or waist circumference. Turns out that drinking diet soda was just as "bad" (or good) as drinking carbonated water.[4]

Recently, scientists took it a step further. They wanted to see if there was any relationship between noncaloric sweeteners (like stevia, Splenda, or aspartame) and a myriad of things like eating behavior, cancer, cardiovascular disease, kidney disease, mood, behavior, and cognition.

They conducted a meta-analysis of fifty-six studies, including twenty-one controlled trials.[5] (A meta-analysis examines a large number of independent studies and is generally considered a stronger standard of evidence.) Once again, they found no negative health impact. Many nutritionists might claim that artificial sugar causes you to gain weight, disrupts insulin, or affects your gut health. But, so far, every time researchers test for those side effects, the claims simply don't play out in real life. When reviewing fifty-six different studies, the researchers found:

- People who consume artificial sweeteners don't have a higher body weight than those who avoid them.
- Using artificial sweeteners doesn't increase hunger or lead to overeating.
- There was no increased risk of cancer.

I don't love to eat artificially sweetened foods, but I can see their value. As you know, obesity is associated with primary causes of death like heart disease, cancer, and diabetes. Artificial sweeteners don't have health benefits, but if you have them every now and then, you can rest assured they won't be damaging your body or making you more prone to weight gain. And, if they're replacing a worse habit, then that can lead to better health outcomes. Let's say someone drinks three regular colas per day. It's not a great habit, so to try to spark positive change, this person swaps out their three regular colas for the diet version. I'm not saying the three diet colas are necessarily healthy (more like health neutral), but those three regular colas per day would equal approximately 50,000 extra grams of sugar per year. The impact of those 50,000 grams of sugar on weight and health is exponentially more than the impact of drinking diet soda. Do the math: multiply 50,000 grams times 4 calories (the amount in a gram of sugar). That's 200,000 calories. Divide that by 3,600 calories (which is the equivalent of 1 pound of body fat) and you get 55 pounds! That's 55 pounds you'd add or keep on your frame with a three-cola-a-day habit. If you switched to artificially sweetened diet soda, you'd lose or never gain those pounds (at least from the soda).

YES, "GOOD" SUGAR DOES EXIST!

We encourage children to eat fruit all the time; we know it's a healthy choice for them. But many adults stay away from fruit because—you guessed it—it contains sugar. Where's the logic in that? Let me make this perfectly clear: there is *no evidence* that eating fruit—even in large amounts—will harm your health.

Look at the research, and there's a lot of it; it's overwhelmingly apparent that fruit helps with weight loss and it's good for general health as well. One study of five thousand Australians found that people who eat fruit daily are about 10 percent less likely to be obese. What's more, another study found that people who are obese or overweight who eat fruit are more successful at losing weight.

Keep in mind that is whole fruit, not fruit juices. Whole fruits are loaded with fiber from their skin and seeds and have substantial water content. Apples, although solid, are 10 percent sugar and 85 percent water, which makes them very hard to overeat. Whole fruits also contain many vital micronutrients that boost overall health. Note that the benefits of fiber and micronutrients are mostly lost during the process of creating fruit juice.

When you eat whole fruits, you are creating an environment in your body that will keep you fuller for longer and will trigger hormones that will make you feel less hungry. There has been a lot of research devoted to determining what happens if you eat a piece of fruit before a meal, and time after time, studies have found that the addition of fruit before a meal helps you eat less of what's on your plate. Some recent studies have also shown that whole fruits may help regulate blood sugar.[6]

The health benefits of fruits are undeniable, but there is yet another reason to reach for fruit whenever you can: its energy density. Energy density refers to how full a food makes you feel given the number of calories. In general, you want to limit foods that have high energy density, meaning you can eat a small amount of the food and take in a lot of calories. The foods you want to eat do the opposite and allow you to eat more volume but with fewer calories. Like fruits!

Adding fruits to your diet is not only beneficial to your health but to maintaining a healthy weight. A high fruit intake leads to a lower risk of obesity. Fresh fruit is ideal when it comes to satiety because of its high water and fiber content and low caloric density.

Years ago, I remember reading an article about how a fruit swap can make a dramatic difference on the scale. As an example, the author explained that if you were to replace a blueberry muffin just one day per week with one cup of blueberries, you would save approximately 20,000 calories per year. That's just one muffin per week. I think the article stuck with me because it highlights the importance of balance. The plan wasn't to get rid of blueberry muffins altogether or suggest that they were permanently off-limits; the idea was to intentionally make healthy swaps in the diet (when possible) by favoring the whole version of something you like instead of a processed version of it.

The blueberry muffin for blueberries swap is a good example, but let's go further. Imagine what would happen if you replaced a calorically dense food with fruit—even if it was only one day a week? Let's say you have a glass of orange juice with breakfast every day. If you ate an orange instead, you would gain the benefits of fiber in the whole fruit and avoid the spike in blood sugar you can get from the high-sugar, low-fiber content of the juice.[7] By making these kinds of swaps, you could still enjoy the less-healthy option on occasion while at the same time cut potentially hundreds or thousands of calories from your diet, feel fuller, and be more in control of your choices and outcomes.

When you do add fruit to your diet, fresh whole fruit is the way to go! Check out this comparison between fresh and dried fruit. Options other than fresh are simply not as healthy.

Fresh apple, 1 cup	Dried apple, 1 cup
67 calories	210 calories
10 grams of sugar	60 grams of sugar

If you have wondered if it's possible to eat too much fruit, science has the answer. One study investigated what happens when you go crazy adding fruit to your diet. Participants were analyzed to find out what happens when they ate twenty servings of fruit per day.[8] I enjoy fruit, and I don't think I could eat that much. Yet, that fruit binge had no negative effect on weight, blood pressure, or triglycerides (a type of fat). In fact, the participants reduced their LDL cholesterol.

If a sweet craving hits, go for the whole fruit!

MY FAVORITE FRUITS

All fruits are good for you, but some fruits are better for you than others. I prefer to judge fruits by their fiber content.[9] Blueberries, raspberries, blackberries, strawberries, cranberries, and many others are also relatively lower in sugar.

FRUIT	SERVING SIZE (GRAMS)	TOTAL FIBER (GRAMS)*
Raspberries	1 cup (123)	8.0
Pear	1 medium (178)	5.5
Apple, with skin	1 medium (182)	4.5
Blackberries	1 cup (6.8)	8.3
Orange	1 medium (140)	3.0
Strawberries	1 cup (144)	3.0

*Rounded to the nearest 0.5 gram

Some fruits, like grapes, dates, mangoes, watermelons, and pineapples, have relatively higher levels of sugar, so while I definitely eat them on occasion, I try to limit my consumption of these fruits.

The bottom line? As you work to cut added, processed sugar, there's no need to cut out fruit. Enjoy it, and it will likely play a big role in supporting your weight loss as well as supplying your body with many vital nutrients.

The way I am encouraging you to eat is not only a flexible one but walks a middle path that allows you to continue working toward your weight-loss and health goals without veering dramatically from one extreme to another. It's all about sustainability, flexibility, and enjoyability. In the next chapters, you'll learn more about the PATH plan, how to put it together, and (most important) how to make it work for you.

PART II

Putting It All Together

CHAPTER 8

Personalizing Your PATH

Now I'd like to show you how balancing your diet and embracing a variety of foods can make you healthier than ever. The trick is to not get caught up in what you can't eat, but in what you can. When I first started working with my client Jenny, what confused her most wasn't any dietary changes I asked her to adopt; it was something I never mentioned at all. Unlike some of the people who reach out to me, Jenny is very open about her past struggles with food. And while she had made incredible strides on her own, she wanted my help with creating more structure in her diet and introducing more balance to what she was eating.

IS IT CHEATING?

After a few weeks of working together, she was doing great. She was following my eating plan, which focused on her eating more fibrous carbohydrates and lean proteins while trying to cut back on added sugars. I quickly discovered that Jenny really enjoyed preparing her own meals. Once I gave her a dozen very simple recipes that she could master, it not only boosted her confidence about what she could cook but also gave her a feeling of control over her food intake.

There was one thing Jenny ate that was not part of any of the recipes or eating plans that I had given her. She was very honest and told me that, usually after dinner, she needed to eat chocolate. It wasn't anything excessive. Maybe a few squares, at most, but it was her nightly indulgence. After she told me, I didn't say anything more about it. A few weeks later, she brought up the post-dinner chocolate again and wondered why I hadn't said something, because she was sure what she was doing was wrong.

"I'm confused. Every day you comment on my food choices and give me feedback. You tell me that I can eat more carbohydrates, or I can drink more water. But you never comment on my eating chocolate. Are you waiting for me to say something?"

She was caught off guard when I asked, "Do you enjoy it?" Not surprisingly, she said, "Yes." My follow-up question was, "Do you feel you could eat this way for the rest of your life?" Again, she said, "Yes."

I explained there was no reason for her to stop eating the chocolate or for me to mention it because a good diet is built around eating nutrient-dense options the majority of the time. When you do that, you naturally create room for foods that are designed solely for satisfaction. (Remember my chocolate chip cookie?) Those small chocolate squares are a net positive for Jenny because they bring her joy and make her feel like she has freedom in what she eats. Joy and freedom are two of the most valuable aspects of a healthy, sustainable, and successful diet.

Good nutrition isn't solely about eating in a way that teaches you what foods to eat for the impact they have on your mind and body. Although food is fuel, it serves other valuable roles. It is possible to appreciate the foods that make you lean and strong just as much as those that simply make you smile because you love them, and they taste good.

Chocolate is Jenny's thing. Mind you, Jenny isn't scarfing down an entire chocolate cake or an extra-large bag of candy. She's having a few squares of dark chocolate as a treat that doesn't take the place of anything else in her diet. You may have something you like that probably isn't included in your average weight-loss plan. There might not be anything special about your choice of chocolate or cookie or snack, but there is something important and satisfying about it for you. Personalizing your diet with what works best for you and fits within your plan creates a little bit of magic that can give your diet the lasting power it needs.

LEARNING FROM PAST MISTAKES

If you want to plot a better future, it helps to study the lessons from your past. To know what will work for your body, you need to honestly assess what has not worked in previous diets so you can determine where things went wrong and why. Then you will be able to focus on the good—those things that were easy or helped you stay on course—and leave the bad behind, which typically includes extreme restrictions and impossible-to-follow advice.

For many people, the idea that they can never eat a certain food again is enough to set off cravings and drive those people to break their new diet plan immediately. When you allow yourself a small indulgence, that can pave the way for keeping you on the road to health and weight loss. Jenny's chocolate is important to her because that tiny splurge, which she chose, allowed her to remain healthy while following a nutritious plan that was designed to help her lose weight. The diet works without the chocolate, but it's less likely to work for Jenny. No matter how balanced or nutritious the diet is, for Jenny, without the chocolate, everything else falls apart.

Most people start their weight-loss quest by asking, "What can get me the quickest results?" Unfortunately, this perspective leaves you vulnerable to the typical downfalls of diet culture and can set you up to fail. When you focus only on results, you may fall for the hype about a plan or program that calls for strict eating or eliminating certain nutrients, and promises quick weight loss in return.

However, when you start your weight-loss journey from a perspective of "How can I make this new, healthy eating plan last as long as possible?" you're setting yourself up for success. When you take the long view, it allows you to factor in your personal needs and preferences that can help you stay with this way of eating for the long haul.

People often have a hard time believing that you can make almost any diet work and still be able to go beyond the parameters of the diet. I'm not talking about modifying a diet due to health requirements like avoiding gluten if you have celiac disease or peanuts if you have an allergy. I am talking about nonmedical needs and personal preferences that can help you keep on track: for example, "I enjoy having pasta with my family sometimes" or "I have to eat dessert." Whether you're a carb lover or chocoholic, just like Jenny, the flexibility of filling your plate by following PATH will help you to make it work for your weight-loss and health goals.

BUILDING A DIET PLAN THAT MEETS *YOUR* NEEDS

If losing weight and being healthy were as simple as eating whatever you want, no one would be frustrated by dieting because no one would need a diet in the first place. With some work and a bit of trial and error, it is possible to build a diet plan that meets your needs, prevents weight gain, and helps you lose fat and acquire muscle. The best diet plan is a by-product of a little "give and take." You figure out what you must take (your personal needs or requirements) and then balance that out by giving in other ways (giving up some of the things—like excess sugar and added fats—that may be keeping you from achieving your diet and health goals).

The essential components for a diet that works, like *The Carb Reset*, are found in the optimal ratio of carbohydrate, protein, and fat. We know that both high-fat and high-carb diets can be effective for any weight-loss goal. But you can't have a large amount of these nutrients at every meal. This is where the concept of "dietary balance" comes into play. Here's how it works: Let's say you love pasta. Because pasta is a carb-heavy meal, you need to make sure you balance it out with a similar amount of protein, a little bit of fat, and often some added fiber. If done correctly, the total number of calories you consume will be on point without restricting a food you love. I have plenty of clients who can eat pasta every week, even when they are trying to lose a lot of weight. My job isn't to restrict the foods they love; it's to adjust what they put on their plate at every meal to make it work for them.

That same balance can be brought to movement and exercise. If you do what you love—rather than what you think you have to do—you can avoid burning out and be much more consistent. You don't need to commit to doing Instagram-worthy, crazy-intense workouts. Simply try to do more of the activities that you enjoy and incorporate them into your daily life.

WHAT DO YOU WANT TO ACHIEVE?

To know where you are going and put yourself on the right path to get there, you need to have a clearly defined destination in mind. It's worth taking the time to dial in to what you truly want to achieve so you can not only have a result in mind but also be able to mark your progress along the way.

If you are trying to lose weight, do you have a certain number of pounds in mind? Or do you want to drop some weight so you can feel a certain way? Is your current weight standing in the way of your performing a specific activity? Maybe you want to lose pounds and inches so you can fit into a favorite pair of jeans? To find goals that are specific to your life and what you want to get from following a new eating plan, you can use the SMART technique.

THE SMART TECHNIQUE

SMART stands for: Specify, Measure, Action, Responsible, Time. I will break it down for you so you can apply it to setting goals for weight loss and health. A bonus of becoming familiar with the SMART technique is that you can apply it to any goal you'd like to achieve. Let's look at how it can be applied to your diet. You can write down your goals in a notebook to help keep them front of mind and monitor your progress.

1. Specify

What is it that you're trying to accomplish? Saying "lose weight" is not specific enough. The more specific your goal is, the better—for example, "I want to lose fifteen pounds in six months." Whatever the goal, declare it so you know where you are headed and can then determine how to get there.

2. Measure

Determine how you are going to measure your goal. You need to be able to assess your progress, but don't do it in a way that will invite obsession or cause you to abandon the plan. Strictly relying on the numbers on the scale isn't the best approach. Remember, body weight can be deceiving, so it's good to have different ways to measure your progress. For example, if your weight stayed the same but your clothes fit better, and you lost inches and your body fat decreased, that means you lost fat (and probably a lot of it) and that's a win! Make sure you know what success looks like (and it might be different from what you expect).

3. Action

You can choose from many different actions to begin your journey to success. For example, you might start with a goal for increasing your weekly steps (be sure you have a number attached to it to make it measurable), increasing the amount of fiber-rich carbs you add to your plate, or how much sleep you get each night. When you make these targets actionable, you give yourself an opportunity for success. Be sure that they facilitate making changes but are reasonable. If they are too far out of reach, you may set yourself up for failure, become frustrated, and quit before you've started. Whatever action you decide to take, focus on doing it for a time until it feels easy to achieve. As you reach your incremental goals, you can build on them—add more steps, eat more carbs, gain more sleep. Take it step-by-step and keep in mind that the actions you take could change over the course of working toward a goal.

4. Responsible

Who will help keep you on track? Change is hard, but it becomes less difficult when you can share and celebrate your successes or get support when you are struggling with your goals. Having a system in place to hold yourself accountable is essential. You could follow the PATH eating plan with a friend and give support to each other. You can hold yourself accountable and make a note of what you intend to do on your calendar, set up reminders on your phone, or use whatever you need to keep yourself on track.

5. Time

Most weight-loss goals aren't unrealistic; they simply follow an unrealistic timeline. Set goals so that you don't get easily discouraged. Keep in mind that healthy weight loss often means one to two pounds per week. This may not seem like much, but when you apply this rate of weight loss to a goal of losing fifteen pounds in six months, you would achieve your goal long before the six months was up. That said, diets have plateaus—times when you may find you are not losing weight or not losing at the same rate—and that needs to be factored in to your goal and timeline setting. Many people see a plateau as a failure when it is simply part of the natural progression of weight loss. If you don't see change in a given week, you can assess if you have gone off your plan in some way and take corrective action, but you will more than likely realize that you are doing just fine. Stick with it, and don't let a perceived "failure" prevent you from staying on track.

WHAT *HASN'T* WORKED FOR YOU?

Knowing what doesn't work is nearly as important as knowing what does. However, I'm going to encourage you to let go of feeling bad about past "failures." At some point, everyone has tried to change the way they eat and not seen the results they wanted. Success is about adjustments. Those diet misfires are great teaching tools that will inevitably help you discover solutions that will work for you. Before you can change your future, you need to ensure you don't fall for the same mistakes that caused you trouble in the past. In many cases, "failure" comes from trying to do too much too soon and pursuing severe restrictions, which often lead to giving up.

I recommend that instead of trying to completely overhaul your lifestyle, you first take an honest look at it. For better or worse, the habits that are a part of your daily schedule won't be easy to change immediately. When you want to change how you eat, trying to change everything all at once is likely, no pun intended, biting off more than you can chew. It is more than possible to change your behaviors and you will get healthier—but it will take some time. So the best approach is to keep the big-picture changes of *The Carb Reset* in mind, but remember that you shouldn't try to change everything all at once. Taking small steps in the right direction can get you where you ultimately want to go.

MAKING ADJUSTMENTS TO YOUR MEALS THAT WORK

As stated previously, one of the key tenets of *The Carb Reset* is that there are no foods that are off-limits, no foods that you can *never* eat, and essentially no "bad" foods. However, there are guidelines on the quantities of foods to eat at each meal (the PATH approach), as well as about the choices you can make to fill your plate in a way that leaves you full but also reaching and maintaining your weight-loss goals.

TAKE A GOOD-BETTER-BEST APPROACH

Using PATH to fill your plate helps you to adjust your carbs along with the fats, veggies, and proteins you eat to keep you on track. Another helpful tool is what I call the good-better-best continuum. It's a hierarchy you can use to make upgrades for just about any type of food.

For example, if you love eating bread, you could think of white bread as level 1 ("good"), 100% whole wheat bread at level 2 ("better"), and a seeded sourdough at level 3 ("best"). These sorts of switches won't necessarily reduce your calorie intake, but choosing better or best over good is a pathway to eating more nutrient-dense foods that might provide additional satiety (the feeling of fullness), which could ultimately help you eat a little less. Notice I'm not calling white bread "bad." It's just that it's not nutrient-dense, so it doesn't carry as many health benefits as other options do and it won't fill you up like other forms of bread that are loaded with fiber.

Making more substitutions for the best version doesn't mean you have to completely go without the good versions. If you're a carb lover, find one meal per day that you're more likely to indulge in the good carb options. This might be pancakes at breakfast, a sandwich on white bread at lunch, or pasta at dinner. You can change the meal you emphasize each day. When you have a meal that features a good carb, then the rest of your meals that day should consist of lean proteins (your choice of fish, meat, chicken, plant-based sources, or others), vegetables, fruits, and some fats like nuts, seeds, or olive oil. Eating this way provides daily flexibility so that you're not engaging in restriction but building the good habits (eating more protein and vegetables, for example) that are the foundation of any successful diet plan.

EAT ON YOUR TERMS

Your job isn't to eat on someone else's schedule; it's to eat when you're hungry. Many people wake up in the morning and say that they don't feel hungry but crave food at night. Others get up and immediately feel famished but don't desire as much food in the evening. Both "craving" cycles—and anything in between—can be satisfied by following completely different approaches. In the meal plan section (see chapter 10), you'll see that you have options for three meals per day plus snacks. But, within those guidelines, it's important not to overthink when you eat.

1. Don't Stress Breakfast Timing

I love breakfast. I think it is a valuable meal because you've gone many hours without ingesting any nutrients. Your blood sugar is low, and your body is in a muscle-wasting (catabolic) state because you haven't had protein. But just because I'm a big believer in breakfast doesn't mean you need to stress over how early you consume your first meal of the day. You don't have to eat the moment you wake up and you don't have to arbitrarily wait hours before you eat either. If you're not a big breakfast person, I suggest you start the morning with something small like nonfat Greek yogurt with berries or an apple with a couple slices of fat-free cheese. A small snack can give your body some good nutrition to start your day—a good, healthy habit.

BENEFITS OF BREAKFAST

1. **REDUCED RISK OF OBESITY:** People who regularly eat breakfast are 30 percent less likely to be obese compared with those who skip breakfast.[1]
2. **IMPROVED METABOLISM:** Eating breakfast kick-starts your metabolism early in the day, leading to better energy expenditure throughout the day.[2]

3. **BETTER NUTRIENT INTAKE:** Breakfast eaters tend to have higher intakes of essential nutrients like vitamins and minerals, which are crucial for overall health.[3]

4. **ENHANCED COGNITIVE FUNCTION:** Breakfast consumption has been linked to better cognitive performance, including memory and concentration.[4]

5. **STABLE BLOOD SUGAR LEVELS:** Eating breakfast helps regulate blood sugar levels, reducing the likelihood of insulin resistance and type 2 diabetes.[5]

These studies underscore the importance of having a nutritious breakfast as part of a healthy lifestyle, contributing to both weight management and overall well-being.

---

2. Snack Smarter

I also think that eating more than three meals per day is beneficial, but not necessary. I think it is better when people eat proactively rather than reactively. I recommend snacks between meals because if you become too hungry, it is likely that you will then eat in a way that doesn't support smart, healthy eating. You could find yourself eating too much of the foods that appeal more to your taste buds (salty, sugary, fatty) than will support *The Carb Reset* approach to healthy eating. Although the grazing method (eating five or six smaller meals or snacks) was all the rage for many years because of theories about how it would boost your metabolism, those theories turned out to be misleading because multiple meals throughout the day do not have a significant impact on metabolism. The real reason that snacking and eating smaller meals works is that the practice keeps hunger at bay and allows you to make better choices about what you are eating when you do sit down for a meal.

SMART SNACKING

Research on snacking and weight loss tends to focus more on the quality and timing of snacks rather than advocating for snacking itself as a weight-loss strategy. However, here are five points that highlight how snacking can potentially support your weight-loss efforts:

1. **IMPROVED APPETITE CONTROL:** Careful and planned snacking can help reduce feelings of hunger and prevent overeating at main meals. For example, consuming a high-protein snack between meals has been shown to increase satiety and reduce subsequent food intake.[6]

2. **MAINTAINING METABOLIC RATE:** Eating small, frequent meals (including snacks) throughout the day can help maintain a stable metabolic rate, which may support weight loss by preventing your metabolism from slowing down.[7]

3. **BALANCED BLOOD SUGAR LEVELS:** Healthy snacks that include a combination of protein, fiber, and healthy fats can help stabilize your blood sugar levels, reducing cravings and the likelihood of consuming high-calorie snacks.[8]

4. **ENHANCED NUTRIENT INTAKE:** Nutrient-dense snacks such as fruits, vegetables, nuts, and yogurt provide essential vitamins, minerals, and antioxidants, supporting overall health and potentially reducing the risk of weight gain.[9]

5. **BEHAVIORAL CONTROL:** Planning and consuming healthy snacks can promote mindful eating and help you make better food choices throughout the day, leading to improved weight management outcomes.[10]

These studies emphasize that while snacking itself may not directly cause weight loss, strategic snacking can play a supportive role in a balanced diet aimed at weight management and overall health.

The best approach to effective snacking is to make sure that you are in control of how much you eat (note that the portion of "snacks" has nearly tripled in size in the last twenty years) and be sure that you are eating only when you're hungry, and not just because you feel like you need to sneak in another meal. Some people snack because they are legitimately hungry and prefer to eat smaller portions spaced throughout the day. Other people fall victim to snacking triggers like frustration or boredom. To put your snacking in perspective, your first step is to examine what's setting off your snack attacks.

Another thing to pay attention to is how much you are really snacking. A snack that staves off hunger before your next meal is okay; mindless munching is not. For example, let's say you're supposed to spread a tablespoon of peanut butter on some apple slices. The reality: you wind up spooning almost half the jar of peanut butter directly into your mouth, and the apple *might* get eaten as an afterthought. Or, perhaps you're supposed to eat a serving of hummus with some veggies. Without really noticing what you've been eating, you realize the whole tub of Sabra is empty, because after the veggies disappeared so quickly, you broke out a bag of tortilla chips to help finish it off. (After all, it's a snack, right?)

When these "supposed tos" are difficult to execute because the servings are so small, or the suggested foods just aren't satisfying, you are set up to fail. So if you find yourself standing on the scale in disbelief that the number hasn't shifted, or wondering why your pants are tighter, you may find yourself thinking:

- *"I don't know why I'm not losing weight (or am actually gaining pounds) because I'm not technically eating anything bad."* You are frustrated because you are eating the "right" foods but not getting the "right" results.
- *"Why can't I just snack like a normal human being? Why am I so weak?"* You're swimming in guilt with bouts of overeating that you can't control.

This is a common problem. In fact, you're no different from most people who have some trouble figuring out how to make healthy snacks work for their meal plan or to rein in overeating.

So if you're someone who's more likely to chow down when you're bored, I recommend that you clear your kitchen and cupboards of pre-packaged foods—if it's there and handy, you are more likely to eat it. Meanwhile, if you're someone who gets hungry often and finds yourself eating several smaller meals throughout the day, then protein may be your friend when it comes to keeping weight off. Research shows that snackers who switched to high-protein foods lost more body fat.[11]

I'm a huge proponent of three meals and two snacks per day, but I realize that might not work for everyone. Some people don't have time, or prepping five meals a day feels stressful. Bottom line, try eating three meals and one snack daily. See how that works for you, and if you are still hungry, feel free to add a second snack.

3. Satisfy Your Sweet Tooth

If you have a sweet tooth, there are several ways to help satisfy your craving (or break the habit, if you wish). These recommendations aren't mutually exclusive, so feel free to use elements of each.

OPTION #1: CREATE BOUNDARIES—If you have trouble controlling how much you eat, try to have sweets only outside your home. This means you can enjoy ice cream with a friend at your favorite spot, but you can't buy a carton of ice cream and stash it in the fridge. Out of sight, out of mind—or at least, out of easy access.

If you share your living environment, or you entertain a lot and as a result have sweet snacks on hand and aren't able to eliminate all the sugars and sweets from your home, then consider option #2.

OPTION #2: DOWNSIZE—Buy smaller-size portions of the packaged sweets you have on hand. The smaller size helps enforce portion control. Research shows that portion sizes have expanded over the years.[12]

In some cases, the change is massive, such as burgers being 50 percent larger than they were in the 1970s. When you choose the larger portion sizes, research suggests that you could eat 30 percent more calories per day. This might seem obvious, but, in that same research, only 45 percent of people noticed they were overeating.

Often the issue isn't *what* you eat but rather *how much*. If you reduced the portion sizes of the foods you need to limit (like those loaded with added sugar or saturated fats), you would take a significant step forward in improving your health.

OPTION #3: REPLACE—Can you swap your favorite guilty pleasure with something that hits on the same notes in terms of flavor and texture? I love smoothies because when a sweet craving strikes, I can drink a cool, creamy, fruity creation instead of turning to a calorie-loaded dessert. Cravings are a challenge, but I want you to learn how to embrace them rather than run from them, because the more you try to avoid them, the more likely you are to give in—and potentially overindulge. Approaching food cravings by finding healthier substitutes makes it much less likely that you'll feel deprived and stressed—at a time when your healthy behaviors are most likely to completely fall apart.

PREPARE FOR LIFE ON THE GO

I've worked with many people who are "on" from dawn to dusk and don't always have the time to cook. If you are strapped for time to prepare meals, the trick is to have something healthy that you can make relatively quickly, and then enjoy repeatedly throughout the week. In this case, spending just a little bit of time on snack prep can help set you up for success. Pick one or two recipes that you cook once but can enjoy several times. In other words, cook with leftovers in mind.

I have a pretty busy schedule (probably just like you), so on Sunday I take time to plan ahead and prevent meal prep stress. Every

Sunday morning, I take my kids to the local farmers' market. We go to the fruit and vegetable stand and get bell peppers, spinach, and berries. We visit the fish market and buy salmon and shrimp. We spend time together selecting fresh foods that we love. That night, while my kids are playing, I spend about an hour of cathartic meal prep of foods that I intend to use over the next few days. While some salmon is in the air fryer, I steam broccoli and grill shrimp. I blend my broccoli into soup and prep veggies for snacks. After an hour, I've got food covered for the whole family for the next four or five days. I always have healthy food choices available so I can eat quickly when I'm hungry, so I don't risk ordering takeout or eating an entire bag of chips. Setting myself up for success helps me stay on track, and it will work for you, too.

If meal prep isn't your thing, you can strategically make bigger portions and turn every meal into two meals. When you make dinner at night, double the portion size. Before you serve the food, take half and store it in your fridge. This becomes your lunch for the next day. These meals don't have to be complex; they can be simple, like tacos made from some grilled or sautéed vegetables; add a source of protein, and you're good to go.

When you build a diet to fit your life (rather than trying to do it the other way around), you're in the driver's seat on the road to positive change. That alone can make a huge difference to your success.

THREE HABITS THAT DRIVE RESULTS

Changing from doing what you've always done to living the way you want takes adjustment. Honestly, not having that adjustment period is where some other diets you've probably been on have failed you. You can't overhaul your diet overnight, but you can make thoughtful trade-offs that allow you to adapt to a new way of eating. It's okay to continue to eat some of your old favorites while at the same time adopting new foods that will keep you moving toward your goals. Once you get the hang of eating in a new way, you'll be eating with the flexibility that will make it easier to succeed. It all begins with healthier behaviors that are easy to replicate. You can build your foundation with some simple habits that prevent you from losing your way.

Habit #1: Embrace Quality Calories

When I was at university, I learned how high-volume, low-energy-dense foods are one of the most effective tools for weight loss. Remember, most diets focus only on restriction and removal. *The Carb Reset* helps you add a variety of foods to your plate. The ratio of macronutrients is critical. I call this way of eating the trinity of satiety—eating more lean protein, fiber, and healthy fat. Research shows that the addition of one, two, or all three of these nutrients improves blood sugar stability and increases satiety. Eating foods in combination as PATH lays out is the key. Rice gets a bad rap, because people obsess over its glycemic index. But they are looking at rice in isolation. In reality, no one sits down and eats a meal of rice. In real life, rice is typically eaten along with fats and protein as well as veggies. That combination of nutrients changes how your body responds to the foods you eat. It's good to consider the glycemic impact of an entire meal, not focus on one ingredient. When you combine the right foods, your blood sugar won't spike, your hunger will be under control, and you'll still have room for dessert and not feel ravenous after you enjoy it. Sounds pretty good, right?

Habit #2: Control Your Cortisol

Cortisol is a hormone associated with weight gain and stress. As your cortisol rises, it increases the factors that contribute to weight gain: your appetite increases; you desire additional sweet, fat, salty foods; and your hunger is less likely to be satisfied.

THE CORTISOL CONNECTION

Cortisol, often referred to as the stress hormone, plays a significant role in metabolism and weight regulation. Here are five factors that demonstrate its impact on weight gain:

1. **INCREASED ABDOMINAL FAT:** Chronic elevation of cortisol levels has been associated with increased abdominal fat. One study found that higher cortisol levels correlated with greater waist circumference and accumulation of visceral fat—fat found deep in the body around the organs, which protects them, but too much can be tied to cardiovascular disease, stroke, and diabetes.[13]

2. **INCREASED APPETITE AND CRAVINGS:** Elevated cortisol levels can lead to increased appetite and cravings for high-calorie foods, particularly those high in sugar and fat. Research indicates that cortisol may influence food intake by altering the activity of brain regions involved in reward and appetite regulation.[14]

3. **IMPACT ON INSULIN SENSITIVITY:** Cortisol can impair insulin sensitivity, leading to elevated blood sugar levels and potentially contributing to the development of insulin resistance and type 2 diabetes. Studies have shown that chronically elevated cortisol levels are associated with insulin resistance and metabolic dysfunction.[15]

4. **DISRUPTING SLEEP PATTERNS:** Cortisol dysregulation, often observed in conditions of chronic stress, can disrupt sleep patterns. Poor sleep quality and duration have been linked to weight gain and obesity, possibly due to changes in appetite-regulating hormones like leptin (the fullness hormone) and ghrelin (the hunger hormone).[16]

5. **IMPACT ON METABOLIC RATE:** High cortisol levels can lead to a decrease in basal metabolic rate (BMR), which is the amount of energy your body needs to maintain basic physi-

ological functions at rest. Lower BMR may make it more challenging to maintain or lose weight.[17]

These studies highlight the complex relationship between cortisol levels, stress, metabolism, and weight regulation, underscoring the importance of stress management and maintaining healthy cortisol levels for overall health and weight management.

Because of the cortisol–weight gain connection, you want to do everything you can to lower your cortisol. Maintaining carbs in your diet is a great start, because consuming too few carbs can increase cortisol. Another way to keep cortisol in check is to limit alcohol consumption, reduce caffeine, and be mindful of your screen time. No, I'm not banning all wine, coffee, and screen time; I'm recommending a *reduction* in the amounts you consume during your day. Because repeated doses of caffeine throughout a day have been shown to elevate cortisol levels, the best approach may be to have your morning joe but pass on the afternoon pick-me-up.[18] Alcohol can also encourage an uptick in cortisol, especially when consumed in a large amount over a short time span. A glass of wine with dinner is probably okay, but having an entire bottle each night will not do your body any favors.

As for your phone and other screens, they might be the biggest cortisol trigger of all. Research published in *Environmental Research* found that "excessive screen time is associated with poor sleep and risk factors for cardiovascular diseases such as high blood pressure, obesity, low HDL cholesterol, poor stress regulation (high sympathetic arousal and cortisol dysregulation), and Insulin Resistance."[19]

In other words, the more time you spend on your phone and other screens, the more likely you are to have a host of health issues or poor behaviors that lead to health problems. We typically think of excessive screen time as the well-publicized troubles linked to social media, but it's also the notifications, work emails, and attachment to electronic devices and how they capture your attention and time. Constantly being connected can trigger stress, and as that stress builds up, cortisol rises and can damage your overall health.

Working on stress reduction can have a life-changing impact on your happiness as well as your hunger. Stress itself can increase cortisol, and the more cortisol rises, the more your stress defense shuts down. Breathing is one of the easiest and most accessible ways to stop stress and elicit a relaxation response.[20] Taking a few deep, controlled breaths can turn your "fight or flight" into "rest and digest."

So the next time you find your mind racing and feel the need to hit the panic button, step away from the computer, put down your phone, find a quiet place, and take a seat. Then spend five minutes doing belly breathing. Sitting with your hand on your belly, take a deep full breath through your nose and feel your belly expand with the breath. Then exhale through your mouth until you feel "empty." Then fill up again with a deep full breath, exhale, and repeat the cycle until you feel relaxed.

HABIT #3: SLEEP YOUR WAY TO HEALTH

Poor or insufficient sleep also increases cortisol production and produces other hormones leading to fat storage. In fact, just a few days of poor sleep changes your hormones in a way that is a fat-loss nightmare. When everything is working well, your body releases fatty acids so they can be burned up and used as energy. Without enough rest, that process shuts down, the fat cells aren't released, and fat storage becomes more likely.

That's not all. Research suggests that even a single night of sleep deprivation can increase your level of ghrelin while decreasing leptin.[21] That combination leaves you ravenous and wanting to eat more food. You may have experienced this on days when you have been sleep-deprived and felt like eating everything in sight.

Do what you can to prioritize sleep. Make a plan. Set reminders in your phone for what time you need to start your bedtime routine so you will get enough sleep. Historically, health professionals advocated that people sleep between seven and eight hours per night. However, in my private practice I have had my clients wear activity/sleep trackers like Fitbit or Oura ring to analyze their quality of sleep. Based on more than fifteen years and 75,000 data points, I advocate for ninety minutes of deep sleep and ninety minutes of REM (rapid eye movement) sleep, rather than a gross amount of sleep. In other words, sleep quality is even more important than sleep quantity. Perhaps it might be helpful to have some context. There are multiple phases of sleep: deep sleep, often associated with restoring your body; REM, associated with brain and cognitive function; as well as light sleep and wakefulness. The more you experience deep sleep and REM, the more effective sleep is in helping you rest and restore.

THE OPTIMIZED LIFE CHECKLIST

I want to encourage you to personalize and streamline your healthy living plan. Below, I've created a list of the principles of the healthiest people in the world. You will notice that these principles are not complicated, and that's by design. Being healthy shouldn't be difficult. In fact, the hardest part about living well is ignoring all the information that suggests you need to do something radical. Keeping it simple will lead not only to success, but to feeling healthier, happier, and leaner than ever.

- **Sleep:** As you just learned, a lack of sleep might be why you overeat, crave junk food, and lack energy.
- **Smile:** It's simple, and it reduces stress.
- **Eat protein, carbs, and fats:** Carbs are okay. They are your best friend in limiting fat storage. Protein will fuel your muscles and keep you full. Healthy fats will supply your brain and hormones with the nutrients they need.
- **Drink water:** A lack of hydration can spark hunger pangs that

trick you into eating when you're not actually hungry but are thirsty.

- **Ignore all detoxes, cleanses, and magic pills:** Save your money. None of these "remedies" does anything other than make your wallet lighter.
- **Have sex:** Do I really need to convince you?
- **Set realistic expectations:** Fat loss occurs in spurts. Most people will lose an average of one to two pounds per week. Some months you might "peak" and lose ten to twenty pounds. But, if you're losing four to eight pounds per month without stressing the week-by-week variance, you're on the right track. If that seems low to you, remember . . .
- **Plateau is part of the process:** It does not mean your body is broken. Healthy weight loss that lasts forever will take months, not weeks. There are exceptions, but play the long game for the most part, and you'll never look back. Because don't forget . . .
- **Rapid weight loss can sometimes lead to rapid weight regain:** It's okay if you lose fat quickly when you're not living in the extremes.
- **Movement and exercise are your friends:** Weight training is great, but so is the simple act of going for a walk. Movement fights stress and builds resilience that will help you along the journey. Choose exercises that you enjoy and do them often. Ideally, at least three times per week.
- **Embrace imperfection with diet, exercise, and even your appearance:** You're human. Off days happen when you don't eat as well as you'd like or move as much as you'd like. Take it as a minor detour and get back on the path as soon as you can. Repeat as needed.

I've seen life-changing results when the above advice is followed. People develop abs, those with chronic diseases become healthier, people in their forties and fifties feel like they have turned back the clock, and everyone enjoys food more than they ever thought possible. The best part? You will be happier.

If you think the above list is too easy, consider how much success you've had with the "complex" plans you've tried, or the "cure-all" plans that have brought you back to square one.

The key to a better diet is balance.

- Balance gives you all the nutrients you need.
- Balance keeps you fuller for longer.
- Balance provides variety that prevents you from getting bored.
- Balance gives you the freedom to eat the foods you love without being miserable.

When things are balanced, you can enjoy what you eat *and* be healthy. And, by using PATH to plan out your balanced, tasty meals, you can enjoy what you eat *and* be healthy, because it's difficult to achieve health without enjoyment being a part of your experience.

CHAPTER 9

Getting Past Roadblocks and Detours

Before we get into the specifics of the meal plans, I want you to take a minute to think about some things that will help you avoid the issues you faced with past diets. You may be psyched to dig in but find yourself worried that this time won't be any different from the others. With some diets that ultimately didn't work out, you probably felt like you knew *exactly* what you were supposed to do and believed that these diets would help you achieve your goals. When the reality didn't quite match up with your expectations, you may have blamed yourself, not the diet, and believed that you failed because you did not have enough willpower to stick with it.

While willpower is often blamed for your getting sidetracked—you just couldn't resist eating, overeating, or consuming unhealthy foods—the thing that actually trips up most people and causes them to break with their eating plan isn't a lack of willpower. It is because they are not aware of their triggers.

UNDERSTAND YOUR TRIGGERS

Everybody has food triggers, which can be physical (when you're tired), mental (when you're stressed), hormonal (especially menstrual cycles), or have to do with the foods you eat (some contain a sugar-salt-fat combo that's engineered to make you want to eat more). The trick to breaking free of overeating is learning your triggers and understanding why they set you off.

If you can better understand your triggers, you can identify them before they take control of your behaviors and sabotage your best efforts to be healthy.

FEELING SAD, DOWN, OR DEPRESSED

It almost feels unfair, but when you're feeling down, your body craves more sweet foods. While it would be convenient if you wanted to eat tons of vegetables when you are sad, unfortunately, your body doesn't work that way.

MOOD AND FOOD

There is a complex interplay between mood and appetite regulation, highlighting both psychological and physiological factors involved.

1. **EMOTIONAL EATING:** Positive moods can lead to increased food consumption due to heightened reward sensitivity; negative moods can also trigger emotional eating, often leading to overconsumption.[1]

2. **HORMONAL INFLUENCE:** Mood fluctuations affect hormone levels, such as those of cortisol and serotonin, which regulate appetite and satiety.[2]

3. **PREFERENCE SHIFTS:** Mood states alter food preferences. For instance, positive moods may increase the desire for indulgent foods, while negative moods might shift preferences toward comfort foods.[3]

4. **METABOLIC EFFECTS:** Stress-induced negative moods can alter metabolism, leading to changes in energy expenditure and storage.[4]

5. **BEHAVIORAL PATTERNS:** Chronic mood disturbances like depression or anxiety can disrupt eating patterns, leading to either reduced or increased food intake, depending on individual responses.[5]

Feeling depressed, meanwhile, can lead to what psychologists call *negative urgency*, a term that describes how people get more impulsive the worse they feel.[6] A study of more than six hundred women showed that those who did impulsive things when they were depressed had also dealt with binge-eating episodes at one point or another.

STRESS AND ANXIETY

Your body responds to stress by kicking off a fight-or-flight reaction that causes the hypothalamus to produce corticotropin-releasing hormone. That's a fancy way of saying it shuts down your appetite. That sounds like a good thing, but the appetite suppression lasts for only a short time. When that stress becomes chronic (as it does when you're worried about things like money, your job, or your marriage), then your body's response changes.[7]

Remember how we talked about eating in a way that limits fat storage? Carbs can definitely help with that, but they are not the only aid to limiting fat storage—hormones play a role as well. When hormones change because of stress, they can influence how you store fat. Your adrenal glands release a hormone (cortisol), which increases your appetite. Your body will also secrete insulin, which promotes not only food intake but fat storage as well.[8] That's where things go from bad to worse and overeating kicks in. Studies show that stress not only causes you to consume more food, it also leads to the desire to select higher-fat (read: higher-calorie) foods.[9] Over time, persistent stress can reinforce this habit and make food cues more rewarding to your brain.[10] Thus, the vicious cycle is set up of you not wanting to eat certain foods but nevertheless being drawn to them and feeling like you have no control over what your mind tells you to crave and then eat.

LACK OF SLEEP

Ever wonder why you seem to crave cheeseburgers after an all-nighter? Contrary to popular belief, overeating from a lack of sleep is not the result of having more available hours to eat. It's because the desire for unhealthy snacks becomes hardwired into your circuitry.

Your body tends to produce more ghrelin when it lacks sufficient rest.[11] And studies have proven that you're driven to want higher-calorie comfort foods when you are tired.[12] Once again, this trigger makes it easier for you to store fat because your sleep deprivation will push you toward foods you might want to limit.

Although a single night of poor sleep can induce these effects, over time the cumulative effect of lack of sleep is even worse.[13] Numerous studies indicate that people who get fewer than seven hours of sleep per night are more likely to be obese.[14]

BOREDOM

This scenario will probably feel familiar: You're at home, there's nothing happening, so what do you do? You go to the kitchen and search for some "entertainment" and then eat it. This happens because people will do anything to escape monotony. One study found that participants inflicted painful electric shocks on themselves just to break up a long period of boredom.[15]

The same study found that bored people who had access to M&M's consumed much more of the candy than those in the control group. Another study found that people struggle with overeating more in response to boredom than to any other emotion.[16]

DISTRACTION

There's a reason why a bag of chips disappears so much faster when you're in front of the TV: memory influences consumption. One meta-analysis of twenty-four studies found that when people aren't looking at the food they eat—those Pringles don't spend a whole lot of time in front of your eyes while your favorite show is on—they eat much (much) more food.[17]

The visual cues we receive when we pay attention to what we eat can help us keep our consumption in check. And while distracted eating, in general, causes an increase in immediate food intake according to the review, the effect grew even larger as the day wore on. People who were distracted during their first meal ate more at their next one. Conversely, a different study found that women who were instructed to pay more attention to their food at a meal snacked less later in the day.[18]

DEHYDRATION

If you're the type of person who finds salty foods irresistible, you may want to try drinking a glass of water before you reach for the bag of chips. Researchers have found that your thirst and appetite for sodium share a lot of the same neural mechanisms.[19] You might not be aware of your "neural mechanisms," but your craving for something (anything) salty might be a sign that you haven't been drinking enough, and if you're even slightly dehydrated, your brain will send stronger reward signals in response to salty food.[20] So when you feed your dehydrated body salty snacks, you end up craving more and more.

TROUBLESHOOTING YOUR TRIGGERS

When you know what triggers to watch for, you can find ways to work around them. As we've mentioned, there are some global triggers that are related to overeating, especially snacking, and veering away from your diet goals. By incorporating these trigger busters into your life, you can stay on task and on target to your health goals.

Sleep: If a lack of sleep is your overeating trigger, make seven to nine and a half hours of shut-eye (per night) a nonnegotiable part of your routine. Schedule your bedtime and wake time for a set hour every day, so that you don't fall into old patterns. Set alarms on your phone if necessary or program your TV to turn off at a certain time. Be sure to factor in time for your bedtime routine.

Dehydration: If you think dehydration might be an issue, drink more water. For some people, this obvious solution may be easier said than done. I suggest buying three reusable water bottles. Put one at your desk where you work, one by your bedside table (or near the TV), and a third in your car. Fill them up each day so you have fresh water at hand. In most cases, not drinking enough water is the result of not thinking about drinking water. By creating a visual reminder (the water bottle), you're more likely to drink more.

Distraction: To address distracted eating, avoid having your meals in front of a TV or a computer. Follow Harvard's *The Nutrition Source* newsletter's recommendations to prevent overeating, and look at the food you're consuming.[21] Also, chew more—increased chewing has been shown to reduce calorie intake.[22]

Too much goodness: Having a pantry full of tasty foods (full of salt, sugar, and fat) is setting yourself up for failure. Time for a kitchen makeover. Clean that junk out of your cupboards and you'll be better positioned to succeed. Or, simply put the foods that you desire most (but don't want to completely remove) in an area that you don't visit as often (like a different cabinet in your home). The less you see them, the less likely you are to grab them in a pinch. Out of sight, out of mind.

CARB RESET FAQS

I've been helping people transform their bodies for more than thirty years. During that time, I've been asked hundreds of questions, and I'm sure as you prepare yourself to follow *The Carb Reset* that you have similar ones. I hope the following answers will help provide reassurance and allow you to eat better and improve your life.

What should I expect in the first week?

Consider your first week like an orientation. You will be getting accustomed to new eating habits. It is okay if things aren't "perfect." Keep going. If you can implement the plan with 80 to 90 percent compliance, you should expect to start losing weight immediately. If you don't lose weight, don't panic. Give it one more full week. At the end of that week, assess. If you have not been able to follow the plan, focus on removing obstacles and triggers. Reset and start again.

How do I measure foods that fall into multiple categories? For example, is cheese a protein or a fat?

This is probably the most common question I receive about the PATH method. Most foods don't fit perfectly into one category, and that's okay. There's no need to overthink this because you will be eating foods that are good for you. You can't eat unlimited quantities (other than of veggies), so as long as you're using the PATH guidelines, you're going to be eating the right things in the right amounts. To make your life as easy as possible, and anytime you're unsure of how to categorize a food, use the food lists in this book (see chapter 10).

The following are some of the foods that tend to be the most confusing, and how I categorize them.

- Cheese is primarily a fat. Most cheeses receive far more than 50 percent of their calories from fat. The remaining calories come from a combination of protein and carbohydrates, usually more protein than carbohydrates.
- Peanut butter—or any nut butter, for that matter—is also a fat. Nuts receive 80 to 90 percent of their calories from fat. The remainder comes from a combination of protein and carbohydrates.

- Beans are primarily carbohydrates.
- Leafy greens are part of your vegetable allotment. I mention this because some greens have protein, but you would need to consume such a large amount of a vegetable to get enough protein that it's not worth overthinking.
- Milk can be either a fat or a protein. It depends on whether you're using the whole, 1% or 2%, or nonfat (skim) version. If it's whole milk, then it's mainly a fat source because it receives most of its calories from fat; however, skim or 1% could be considered primarily a protein source, especially some of the newer milks on the market like fairlife, which has 50 percent more protein and 50 percent less sugar than regular milk.
- Plant milks (soy, oat, almond) are similar to milk in that the categorization can vary. But almost all the plant milks, although they have some fat and protein, would be considered a carbohydrate.
- Eggs have protein and fat, but it's best to categorize them as protein.

Do I use my hand measurements before or after I cook and prepare food?

Because this is a method for plating your food, you'll be measuring the cooked or final state. Once your food is ready to eat—whether it's rice, pasta, or chicken—eyeball the size using your hand, and then add it to your plate.

How do I add flavor while keeping calories down?

Use any spices and/or herbs you like when cooking. They are full of flavor, but calorie-free.

Condiments to bump up the taste of your meals may include:

- Mustard (yellow, hot, whole grain)
- Hot sauce
- No-caloric sweeteners like stevia and monk fruit
- Ground cinnamon

- Unsweetened cocoa or cacao powder
- Reduced-sodium soy sauce
- Pesto
- Salsa
- Tamari
- Kimchi
- Sauerkraut

Can I eat more or fewer than three meals and one snack per day?
It is a good idea to eat all your meals and snacks as scheduled during the day—unless you truly are not hungry. Doing so will help you stay satisfied without overly restricting yourself. Eating too little can lead to losing control over your eating habits and eventually ending up in a binge. If you prefer to eat less frequently, you can combine meals and snacks into larger, less-frequent meals. If you prefer to eat more frequently, then you can split your meal into two smaller meals.

Do I have to eat the snack?
No. You do not have to eat a snack if you are not hungry. However, be sure that you aren't avoiding food out of fear of gaining fat. This plan works when you follow it correctly.

What if I am not hungry at mealtime?
It's not necessary to force yourself to eat food if you are not hungry. Follow your hunger cues. Consider pushing your mealtime back an hour and reassess. Or, if you are not able to finish a meal because you are full, wrap the remaining food and save it for later. If you get hungry between meals, return to the food you did not finish. This will keep you on track with your portions for the day.

What if I am feeling hungry between meals?
When in a calorie deficit, experiencing mild hunger from time to time is normal. But it should be manageable, especially if you are eating the right amount of protein and the right type of carbs. To help reduce

hunger, eat plenty of vegetables and lean protein. Vegetables and lean protein have a lot of volume but not a lot of calories, so they make you feel full. Other strategies for overriding those mild hunger pangs include drinking water or clear fluids, chewing gum, distracting yourself (watch a video, play a game on your phone), and going for a short brisk walk.

What about cheat meals?

For those who read my earlier books, you know I don't like the word *cheat*. I prefer to refer to cheat meals as "free meals." The idea of cheat meals can create a bad relationship with food. It sets you up to believe that some foods are good and others are bad, and you are failing if you eat "bad/cheat food." It makes it seem like you're doing something wrong, and it can put pressure on you to be perfect all week—followed by an episode of gluttony. For most people, this cheat meal approach doesn't work and is a slippery slope to including more and more "bad" foods in your diet.

Instead, it's important to know yourself and know what type of "free" approach will work best. Some of you can go six days (or longer) before needing an indulgence. If this is you, then depending on your goals, you might enjoy one or two free meals per week. That means if you have a birthday and date night in the same week, there's no need to stress. You can enjoy both. Other people—like myself—need a small daily treat. That's why I enjoy my cookie or why Jenny enjoys her chocolate. There isn't a single correct approach. This is more about your personality and doing what works best for you.

What about meal timing?

For a weight-loss goal, meal timing is less of a concern than what you are eating during the day. Everyone will be different, depending on your lifestyle, schedule, and preferences, but planning your meals and snacks during the day can help you stay consistent—and successful. If you're eating three meals and two snacks, then you'll be eating roughly every three hours. On your calendar, create a schedule you can follow.

This will make it easier to follow and prevent hunger from finding you. When you can proactively plan when you are eating, you can avoid being overly hungry, be in control of how much you eat, and prevent yourself from consuming too much.

Will eating before bed make me gain weight?

Your weight loss is determined by the number of *total* calories you consume in a day. Period. It doesn't matter what time of day you eat. That being said, some people struggle with certain times of the day when they are more vulnerable to making poor food choices than at other times. If you are someone who is a late-night binger (I assume very few people binge with a chopped salad at midnight), then closing up your kitchen at a certain hour might be helpful to you.

Should I use a food scale?

When you use the PATH approach, you don't need a scale because you have your hand to get balanced portions of food onto your plate.

Can I have coffee?

Yes, but make sure to keep calories down with minimal additions of milk and sugar. In other words, a 300-calorie coffee would be considered a dessert—not coffee. A little cream (or milk) and sugar is okay.

Can I have alcohol?

I believe alcohol might be one of the worst things you can do for your health, in general. It destroys your sleep quality. When you're drinking alcohol, you're also more likely to make poor choices about what to eat and how much you consume. In addition to disrupting your sleep and affecting your eating habits, alcohol has a detrimental effect on your liver's ability to metabolize fat and your kidneys' ability to minimize water retention. I suggest that my clients limit alcohol intake as much as possible. That said, you're a grown-up and you get to do what you want. If you do drink, I suggest you confine yourself to one or two alcoholic beverages per week.

Best: clear liquor with calorie-free mixers (for example, vodka and club soda with a twist of fresh lemon)

Better: Beer with low alcohol by volume (ABV) percentage or red wine

Limit: sugary or salt-laden drinks, drinks with calorie-rich mixers like fruit juices and sodas

What if I don't cook often? Can I have frozen meals?

Yes, of course you can have frozen meals! Sometimes if you are in a rush, you need a convenient option. The biggest issues with frozen meals are usually sodium, calories, and protein. Frozen meals are usually sodium bombs, and they tend to have more than a thousand milligrams of sodium per serving. That's way too much, so look for options with no more than 500 milligrams. As for calories, aim for a meal with 350 to 500 calories, 25 or more grams of protein, and anywhere from 5 to 10 grams of fiber. And don't forget to keep an eye out for added sugar. If you can, try to pick something with less than 5 grams of added sugar per serving.

What about eating at restaurants?

The PATH rules still apply. These days, it's easier than ever to eat healthily at restaurants if you know what you need to have on your plate—and now you do. I say it's easier because you can make almost any food request, right down to changing the items that typically come in an order. Quite often people feel overwhelmed when looking at a restaurant menu. And truth be told, who can blame them? Depending on the restaurant, certain dishes might appear in different languages, include ingredients you've never heard of, and the restaurant might cut corners by adding lots of extra oils, sugars, and salt to make things tastier.

Whenever possible, check out the restaurant menu online before you go. This way you can take your time and decide what you're going to order when you get there, and if nothing catches your eye, perhaps suggest a different restaurant. When you get to the restaurant, first focus on your protein. Are you going to get meat, fish, chicken, vegetable protein? Whatever it is, prioritize that and build around it. Once you've got your protein, make sure you add some vegetables, and then include a fibrous carbohydrate, like rice, quinoa, sweet potatoes, or legumes. Don't be scared to personalize the dish. Ask your server to take it easy on the sauce, or put it on the side, so you can control the amount of sauce or dressing added to your dish.

What about mixed meals or packaged foods where the ingredients aren't clear?

When you are going out, I recommend trying to pick meals that are not combined. For example, at a restaurant, there's no way to easily measure the makeup of a dish like risotto. If you want to use PATH, skip the risotto 90 percent of the time and order foods based on the PATH categories. But once in a while, if you really want risotto, order, enjoy, and don't overthink it. If you typically build your plate the PATH way, and these blended meals are consumed only about 10 percent of the time, it won't have any negative impact on your body. For other foods—specifically ultraprocessed options like French fries or chips— you're going to want to limit how frequently you have them. But, like everything else, that doesn't mean they are completely off-limits. Instead, think of these foods as a combination of your fat source and your carb. You don't want to eat these foods too often because they tend not to be the healthiest sources of these two nutrients, but—again—this is about enabling you to eat and knowing how to stay in control.

Go ahead and grab a palmful, add it to your plate, then load up on protein and vegetables and you're all set!

CHAPTER 10

Kick-Start Two-Week Meal Plan

Hard-and-fast prescriptive diets may sound promising, but they don't work well in the real world, or at least don't work well for long. A typical meal plan tells you *exactly* what to eat, all the time, which means the plan is ultimately limited in how well you can follow it because of its lack of flexibility.

The Carb Reset is super flexible and adaptable to your own taste preferences. I'm going to give you some effective guidelines on how to reframe the way you construct your meals, get familiar with the PATH approach to measuring portions, and give yourself a good solid start on your journey to a healthier body. Consider this to be the most delicious, easy-to-follow prescription you'll ever be given for better health. We're all overworked, overstressed, and have so many decisions to make that deciding what to have for dinner can be enough to make you throw up your hands and head on over to the drive-through. That's the last thing I want you to do. Instead, I'll give you a plan that is simple but has substance.

Fourteen days of meal plans is a great way to start because it's the perfect amount of time to help you retrain your taste buds, establish a better relationship with carbs, and help you nail the exact portions you need to support your goals. When you get to the end of the two weeks, you don't have to abandon these guidelines. They are more than simply a place to start your new way of eating because you can replay these two weeks of meal plans as many times as you like. You can also use them as a guide for eating beyond your two-week kick start. In fact, you can substitute anything in this two-week plan for the recipes that appear in chapter 11. It's also something you can fall back on to guide you if life gets busy and you have trouble figuring out what to eat. In other words, this meal plan is designed to get you started, keep you going, or help you boost your confidence whenever you need to reset, think less, and eat well.

This customized menu is designed to help you burn more fat, support your overall health, and give your body all the nutrients it needs to thrive throughout the day, prevent an afternoon crash, and sleep well at night. From tacos to tuna melts, grilled cheese to burgers, there is something here for everyone. I want you to realize that you can be healthy *and* enjoy what you are eating.

Because of the flexibility built into the plan, you aren't *required* to eat these meals as they are presented. If you find a meal you love, have it as often as you wish. If you don't like it, skip it and substitute in something you enjoy. Following the two-week plan, I've provided a template that will show you how easy it is to build your own meals and mix and match items to create meals that work for you.

THE TWO-WEEK CUSTOMIZED MEAL PLAN

All recipes are found in chapter 11.

WEEK 1

DAY 1

BREAKFAST: **Apple Pie Smoothie (page 142)**

LUNCH: **Turkey Swiss Panini (page 155)**

DINNER: **Poached Salmon with Dill Sauce (page 170)**

SNACK: **Cut veggies and Homemade Hummus (page 190)**

OPTIONAL SNACK: **Handful of almonds (see page 188)**

DAY 2

BREAKFAST: **PB & J Oatmeal Short-Stack Pancakes (page 143)**

LUNCH: **Skillet Grilled Cheese with Tomato Soup (page 156)**

DINNER: **Thai Fusion Taco (page 172)**

SNACK: **Deconstructed Berry Cobbler (page 191)**

OPTIONAL SNACK: **Apple and nut butter (see page 188)**

DAY 3

BREAKFAST: **Chia Seed Pudding (page 144)**

LUNCH: **Tex-Mex Stuffed Baked Potato (page 158)**

DINNER: **Simple Chicken Stir-Fry (page 173)**

SNACK: **Jicama and Lime (page 189)**

OPTIONAL SNACK: **Handful of pistachios**

DAY 4

BREAKFAST: **Baked Apple with Cinnamon Yogurt (page 145)**

LUNCH: **Tuna Melt (page 157)**

DINNER: **Bouillabaisse (page 174)**

SNACK: **Handful of almonds (see page 188)**

OPTIONAL SNACK: **Greek yogurt and bananas**

DAY 5

BREAKFAST: **Spinach and Cheese Omelet (page 146)**

LUNCH: **Anytime Quesadilla (page 160)**

DINNER: **Ratatouille with Grilled Shrimp (page 175)**

SNACK: **Apple and nut butter (see page 188)**

OPTIONAL SNACK: **Cut veggies and Homemade Hummus (page 190)**

DAY 6

BREAKFAST: **Chocolate-Banana Oatmeal Pancakes (page 147)**

LUNCH: **Marinara Pizza Pocket (page 165)**

DINNER: **Veggie Fried Rice (page 176)**

SNACK: **Greek yogurt and berries**

OPTIONAL SNACK: **Edamame (see page 189)**

DAY 7

BREAKFAST: **Broccoli and Cheese Frittata with Avo Toast (page 148)**

LUNCH: **Classic Chopped Salad with Homemade Croutons (page 162)**

DINNER: **Greek Chicken Souvlaki Platter (page 177)**

SNACK: **Cheese and crackers (see page 188)**

OPTIONAL SNACK: **Peanuts**

WEEK 2

DAY 1

BREAKFAST: **Brunch-for-One Mini Quiches (page 149)**

LUNCH: **Five-Minute Wrap (page 163)**

DINNER: **Speedy and Spicy Pasta Arrabbiata (page 179)**

SNACK: **Popcorn (see page 188)**

OPTIONAL SNACK: **Harley Guacamole (page 193) and veggies**

DAY 2

BREAKFAST: **Cereal and berries (see page 141)**

LUNCH: **Burrito (Sweet Potato and Black Bean, page 164, or Salmon Caesar Salad, page 169)**

DINNER: **Chicken Parmesan with Roasted Veggies (page 180)**

SNACK: **Turkey and Pickle Platter (page 189)**

OPTIONAL SNACK: **Deconstructed Berry Cobbler (page 191)**

DAY 3

BREAKFAST: **Sausage, Egg, and Cheese Breakfast Pasta (page 150)**

LUNCH: **Turkey Reuben on Rye (page 161)**

DINNER: **Honey-Mustard Turkey Burger with Oven-Roasted Sweet Potato Fries (page 182)**

SNACK: **Edamame (see page 189)**

OPTIONAL SNACK: **Cut veggies and Homemade Hummus (page 190)**

DAY 4

BREAKFAST: **French Toast with Quick Berry Sauce (page 151)**

LUNCH: **Weekday Turkey Chili (page 166)**

DINNER: **Shrimp Skewers with Parmesan and Pea Fusilli (page 184)**

SNACK: **Apple and nut butter (see page 188)**

OPTIONAL SNACK: **Popcorn (see page 188)**

DAY 5

BREAKFAST: **Veggie Slaw Scramble (page 152)**

LUNCH: **Super-Stuffed Baked Sweet Potato (page 167)**

DINNER: **Chicken Paillard on a Bed of Arugula and Cherry Tomatoes (page 185)**

SNACK: **Handful of almonds (see page 188)**

OPTIONAL SNACK: **Cheese and crackers (see page 188)**

DAY 6

BREAKFAST: **Apple Cinnamon Oatmeal (page 153)**

LUNCH: **Classic Chopped Salad with Homemade Croutons (page 162)**

DINNER: **Bibimbap (page 186)**

SNACK: **Crackers with Smoked Salmon and Herbed (chives) Yogurt (see page 192)**

OPTIONAL SNACK: **Apples and nut butter (see page 188)**

DAY 7

BREAKFAST: **Avocado Muscle Toast (page 154)**

LUNCH: **Burrito (Sweet Potato and Black Bean, page 164, or Salmon Caesar Salad, page 169)**

DINNER: **Easy Chicken Tikka Masala (page 187)**

SNACK: **Harley Guacamole (page 193) and veggies**

MEAL PLAN TEMPLATE AND SAMPLES

Some people love recipes, but I realize that some people don't love, need, or even want to follow a recipe to create their meals. They prefer a simpler approach to mixing and matching foods. If that sounds like you, these meal templates can help. Instead of thinking of everything as a recipe, it allows you to see how you can plug-and-play with endless food options to build the perfect plate without any effort.

Here are visual examples of how to use the PATH plan to create a meal.

SAMPLE MEAL

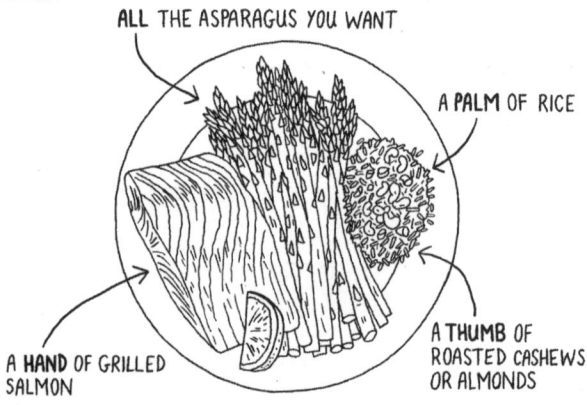

ALL THE ASPARAGUS YOU WANT

A **PALM** OF RICE

A **THUMB** OF ROASTED CASHEWS OR ALMONDS

A **HAND** OF GRILLED SALMON

PROTEIN OPTION: **Fish**
CARB OPTION: **Rice**

FAT OPTION: **Roasted cashews**
VEGGIES: **Asparagus**

SAMPLE MEAL

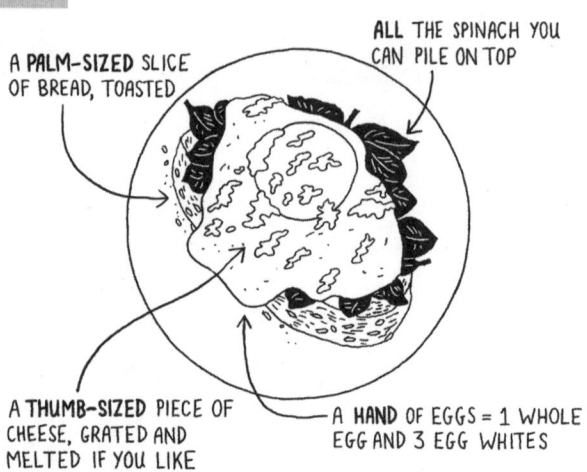

A **PALM-SIZED** SLICE OF BREAD, TOASTED

ALL THE SPINACH YOU CAN PILE ON TOP

A **THUMB-SIZED** PIECE OF CHEESE, GRATED AND MELTED IF YOU LIKE

A **HAND** OF EGGS = 1 WHOLE EGG AND 3 EGG WHITES

PROTEIN OPTION: **1 whole egg and 3 egg whites**
CARB OPTION: **Whole grain bread**

FAT OPTION: **Cheese**
VEGGIES: **Spinach**

SAMPLE MEAL

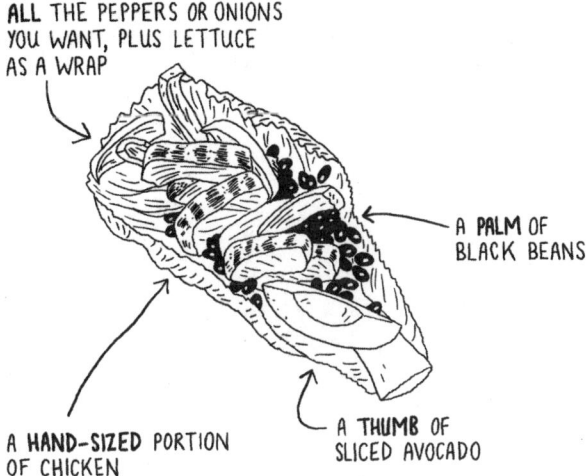

ALL THE PEPPERS OR ONIONS YOU WANT, PLUS LETTUCE AS A WRAP

A **PALM** OF BLACK BEANS

A **HAND-SIZED** PORTION OF CHICKEN

A **THUMB** OF SLICED AVOCADO

PROTEIN OPTION: **Chicken**

CARB OPTION: **Black beans**

FAT OPTION: **Avocado**

VEGGIES: **Bell peppers**

SAMPLE MEAL

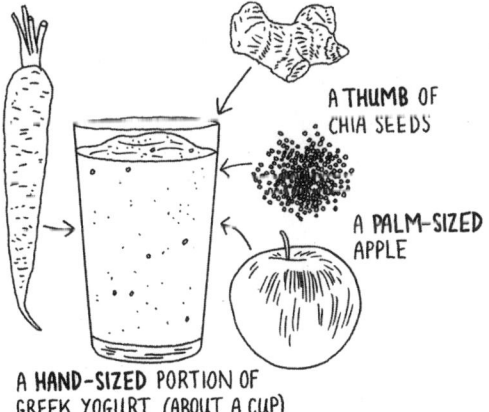

ALL THE CARROTS YOU'D LIKE AND FRESH GRATED GINGER TOO

A **THUMB** OF CHIA SEEDS

A **PALM-SIZED** APPLE

A **HAND-SIZED** PORTION OF GREEK YOGURT (ABOUT A CUP)

PROTEIN OPTION: **Greek yogurt**

CARB OPTION: **Strawberries and blueberries**

FAT OPTION: **Chia seeds**

VEGGIES: **Carrots**

SAMPLE MEAL

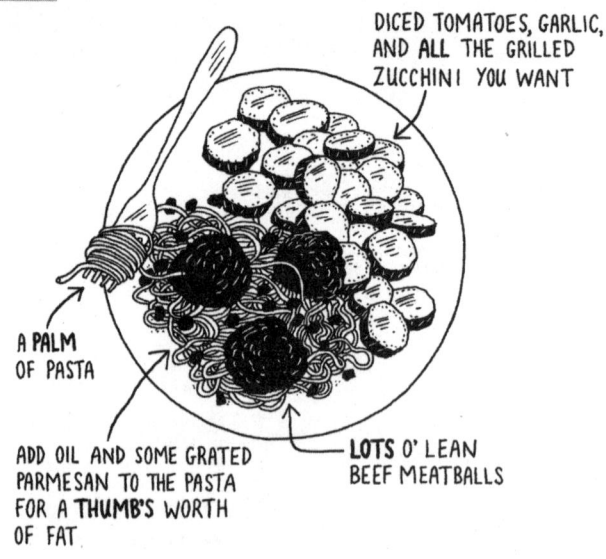

DICED TOMATOES, GARLIC, AND **ALL** THE GRILLED ZUCCHINI YOU WANT

A **PALM** OF PASTA

ADD OIL AND SOME GRATED PARMESAN TO THE PASTA FOR A **THUMB'S** WORTH OF FAT

LOTS O' LEAN BEEF MEATBALLS

PROTEIN OPTION: **Lean beef meatballs**   FAT OPTION: **Olive oil**
CARB OPTION: **Whole wheat pasta**   VEGGIES: **Spinach**

I want to make it as easy as possible to eat in a way that works for you. Each meal follows the PATH approach of combining proteins, carbs, and fat. While this list isn't exhaustive and doesn't contain everything you can possibly consume, it gives you a good idea of how to structure your meals and what types of foods fit within the four different categories found on the PATH plate.

Another option for incorporating this new way of eating into your life is to choose a favorite food from each category and build a customized meal that works for you—that suits your taste buds and fits your schedule. It's a great way to maintain variety in how you eat, but it's also good for developing your go-to favorites that follow the PATH plan.

SAMPLE BREAKFAST

PROTEIN	FATS	CARBOHYDRATES	VEGETABLES AND FRUITS
Chicken (skinless breast or thighs)	Olive oil	Sweet potatoes/Yams	Any green leafy veggie
Eggs (3:1 ratio of whites to yolks)	Nuts (almonds, cashews, Brazil nuts)	Rice (white or brown)	Broccoli
Steak (lean, ground or cuts)	Nut butters	Beans	Spinach
		Whole grains (farro, amaranth, millet, barley, teff)	Arugula
Pork tenderloin	Avocados		Romaine
	Egg yolks	Oats	Brussels sprouts
Turkey (lean, ground or skinless breast)	Seeds (chia, flax)	High-fiber bread/wrap	Asparagus
		High-fiber pasta	Green beans
Greek yogurt			Squash
Nonfat cottage cheese			Kale
			Tomatoes
Whey, casein, egg white, or plant-based protein powder			Celery
			Zucchini
Fish or seafood			Carrots
Tofu			Cucumbers
			Cauliflowers
			Eggplants
			Peas
			Bell peppers
			Grapefruits
			Berries (strawberries, blackberries, raspberries, blueberries)
			Watermelons
			Apples
			Bananas
			Oranges
			Jicama

SAMPLE LUNCH

PROTEIN	FATS	CARBOHYDRATES	VEGETABLES AND FRUITS
Chicken (skinless breast or thighs)	Olive oil	Sweet potatoes/Yams	Any green leafy veggie
Eggs (3:1 ratio of whites to yolks)	Nuts (almonds, cashews, Brazil nuts)	Rice (white or brown)	Broccoli
	Nut butters	Beans	Spinach
Beef (lean, ground or cuts)		Whole grains (farro, amaranth, millet, barley, teff)	Arugula
	Avocados		Romaine
Pork tenderloin	Egg yolks	Oats	Brussels sprouts
Turkey (lean, ground or skinless breast)	Seeds (chia, flax)	High-fiber bread/wrap	Asparagus
		High-fiber pasta	Green beans
Greek yogurt			Squash
Nonfat cottage cheese			Kale
Whey, casein, egg white, or plant-based protein powder			Tomatoes
			Celery
			Zucchini
Fish or seafood			Carrots
Tofu			Cucumbers
			Cauliflowers
			Eggplants
			Peas
			Bell peppers
			Grapefruits
			Apples
			Berries (strawberries, blackberries, raspberries, blueberries)
			Watermelons
			Bananas
			Oranges
			Jicama

SAMPLE DINNER

PROTEIN	FATS	CARBOHYDRATES	VEGETABLES AND FRUIT
Chicken (skinless breast or thighs)	Olive oil	Sweet potatoes/Yams	Any green leafy veggie
Eggs (3:1 ratio of whites to yolks)	Nuts (almonds, cashews, Brazil nuts)	Rice (white or brown)	Broccoli
Beef (lean, ground or cuts)	Nut butters	Beans	Spinach
Pork tenderloin	Avocados	Whole grains (farro, amaranth, millet, barley, teff)	Arugula
Turkey (lean, ground or skinless breast)	Egg yolks	Oats	Romaine
Greek yogurt	Seeds (chia, flax)	High-fiber bread/wrap	Brussels sprouts
Nonfat cottage cheese		High-fiber pasta	Asparagus
Whey, casein, egg white or plant-based protein powder			Green beans
Fish or seafood			Squash
Tofu			Kale
			Tomatoes
			Celery
			Zucchini
			Carrots
			Cucumbers
			Cauliflowers
			Eggplants
			Peas
			Bell peppers
			Grapefruits
			Apples
			Berries (strawberries, blackberries, raspberries, blueberries)
			Watermelons
			Bananas
			Oranges
			Jicama

PERSONALIZING YOUR MEAL PLANS EVEN FURTHER

Many of my clients are vegetarians and you may be, too, and the following chart will help anyone substitute plant-based foods for the (primarily) animal protein in the charts above. In fact, vegetarians may need more protein from plant-based sources because plant proteins are not as "complete" as proteins from animal sources.[1]

VEGETARIAN FOOD SWAP LIST

PROTEIN	FATS	CARBOHYDRATES	VEGETABLES AND FRUITS
Tempeh	Olive oil	Sweet potatoes/Yams	Any green leafy
Tofu	Nuts	Rice (white or brown)	veggie
Seitan	(almonds,	Beans	Broccoli
Textured	cashews,	Whole grains (farro,	Spinach
vegetable/soy	Brazil nuts)	amaranth, millet,	Arugula
protein	Nut butters	barley, teff)	Romaine
Beans,	Avocados	Oats	Brussels sprouts
legumes	Egg yolks	High-fiber bread/wrap	Asparagus
Fish	Seeds (chia,	High-fiber pasta	Green beans
(pescatarian)	flax)		Squash
Plant-based			Kale
protein			Tomatoes
powder			Celery
Nonfat plain			Zucchini
Greek yogurt			Carrots
Nonfat			Cucumbers
cottage			Cauliflowers
cheese			Eggplants
			Peas
			Bell peppers
			Grapefruits
			Apples
			Berries
			(strawberries,
			blackberries,
			raspberries,
			blueberries)
			Watermelons
			Bananas
			Oranges
			Jicama

There are many people who are gluten intolerant—gluten is a protein that is in wheat-based products like breads and pastries. In the following chart, suggestions are given for those who want to avoid gluten and choose what will work for their dietary needs.

GLUTEN-FREE FOOD SWAP LIST

PROTEIN	FATS	CARBOHYDRATES	VEGETABLES AND FRUITS
Chicken (skinless breast or thighs)	Olive oil	Sweet potatoes/Yams	Any green leafy veggie
Egg whites	Nuts (almonds, cashews, Brazil nuts)	Rice (white or brown)	Broccoli
Beef (lean, ground or cuts)	Nut butters	Whole grains (amaranth, teff, buckwheat, millet, polenta)	Spinach
Pork tenderloin	Avocados	Beans	Arugula
Turkey (lean, ground or skinless breast)	Egg yolks	Oats	Romaine
Greek yogurt	Seeds (chia, flax)		Brussels sprouts
Nonfat cottage cheese			Asparagus
Whey or plant-based protein powder			Green beans
Fish or seafood			Squash
Tofu			Kale
			Tomatoes
			Celery
			Zucchini
			Carrots
			Cucumbers
			Cauliflowers
			Eggplants
			Peas
			Bell peppers
			Grapefruits
			Apples
			Berries (strawberries, blackberries, raspberries, blueberries)
			Watermelons
			Bananas
			Oranges
			Jicama

FINDING YOUR COOKIE: YOUR EIGHT-WEEK PLAN TO DAILY DESSERTS

I've mentioned my daily cookie habit and my client Jenny's after-dinner chocolate. I am going to encourage you to find a way to incorporate a daily treat into your life. There's no reason why a treat can't be a healthy habit, and in fact, I think it's part of what makes *The Carb Reset* work.

If a teapot didn't have a steam valve to release the pressure, it would explode. It's similar for us—we can do things a certain way for only so long, without figuratively letting off some steam. A treat serves the purpose of giving you a break, as well as allowing you to eat solely for pleasure. Some people are very binary in their approach to eating and are eating either healthily, or not. Time has shown us that this is not the best approach to supporting and sustaining a way of eating that maintains your health.

I remember when one of my clients canceled our sessions for a week. It turns out they went off to a hardcore diet retreat spa in the desert because they hadn't been eating well for a few weeks, and felt they needed to go away to undo everything they had done to their body. At this ridiculous spa, they ate lettuce and drank lemon water for a week. The program had them do hot yoga and sleep on a bed that felt like a hardwood floor. As soon as they came back from their retreat, they said they felt incredible, had lost weight, and were finally on the right track. Their "success" was short-lived. Within forty-eight hours, they were back to eating the way they were before the retreat, and immediately regained the weight they had lost. As we know, the all-or-nothing approach doesn't get you where you want to go. I encouraged this client to be gentle with themselves when they felt like they hadn't been eating well and slowly reincorporate better eating into their life. There is no need to leave your entire life behind and attend an extreme retreat in the desert to "correct" yourself when you go off track. In fact, because there is room in my plan for an indulgence, I encouraged my client to find their "cookie." Finding your cookie is a helpful way to keep you grounded, allow you to indulge a little, and celebrate food without guilt.

While there are a number of dessert-like options in the Kick-Start Two-Week Meal Plan that you will be enjoying, I want you to find a way to add your preferred treat to your day. The beauty of the treat is that you get to choose what you'd like and add that small daily indulgence to your life. Here's how it works: After the first fourteen days on the PATH plan, I want you to add your preferred treat one day per week. In week 2, add two treats to the week—preferably on two separate days. Then, I want you to continue to add one day of indulgence in weeks 5 through 7. In week 8, you can finally have a small treat every day.

Here's what it looks like:
- **Weeks 1 and 2:** no added treats
- **Week 3:** treat one day per week
- **Week 4:** treats two days per week
- **Week 5:** treats three days per week
- **Week 6:** treats four days per week
- **Week 7:** treats five days per week
- **Week 8:** treats seven days per week

To make this work, I'm going to give you some simple guidelines. First, I want you to avoid the "cheat meal" mentality. That's just another extreme disguised as something good for you when it's probably not. When you follow *The Carb Reset,* the idea is you don't need a break, or need to cheat. You are eating normally, and that includes eating desserts and snacks. That said, I don't want you to go off the rails. A daily treat or snack of your choice is eating one cookie or a few pieces of chocolate. It's not a license to eat a giant donut every day.

That doesn't mean donuts or big slices of cake are totally off-limits. You can eat these treats when it makes sense, such as on a special night out or at a celebration. And if you do eat something like cake or donuts, because you're following *The Carb Reset,* you don't need to make any radical changes to compensate for them. There's no need to fast the next day, detox, or sweat for hours in the gym. You can simply return to your daily way of eating and act like you did nothing wrong—because you didn't.

When treats are normalized, your sugar cravings will decrease. Therefore, you likely won't have cravings and feel like you need those binge-style cheat days. That push to cheat happens when you feel deprived of "forbidden" foods. You know how I feel about too much sugar, and you know it is super tasty, especially combined with fats and so on. So it might take some discipline to reduce sugar in your diet to a small treat, but when you look at the big picture and see that you can have a daily indulgence and it won't "break" your diet, it can help you stick to the overall plan.

Additionally, you can always course correct. For example, if you eat more treats than allotted, repeat the week. For example, if week 4 hits and you have a small treat four times instead of two, don't progress to week 5. Instead, repeat week 4 until you hit the goal.

So much of learning to eat better isn't only stepping away from restrictions and fear, it's also giving yourself the time it takes to adapt to this new style of eating. Don't expect every day to be easy; sometimes you might stumble. But when you do, just continue following the plan, and everything will get easier as you go along.

And, if for some reason you completely fall off the wagon, hit the reset button. Go back to weeks 1 and 2, follow the meal plan, and then build your way back up to having treats. That's the real joy of *The Carb Reset* approach. It's a timeless way to eat. And you can apply it to your life in any situation, scenario, or goal.

CHAPTER 11

The PATH Recipes

When I traveled around the world to do my research for *The 5-Factor World Diet,* a book I wrote many years ago, I noticed that people outside of the United States cook most of their meals at home. Going out to a restaurant was a special event. By cooking food at home, they were able to control exactly what and how much went into each dish. They were familiar with the ingredients and connected to the final dish. Not only is it healthier to eat what you cook but it's far more cost-effective. I wanted to bring this approach to *The Carb Reset* because I know how beneficial it can be.

I realize that cooking can be stressful for many people. They aren't comfortable in the kitchen or don't know how to cook. But I think that the primary barrier to making meals at home is time. People feel crunched for time and need to move quickly from work or school to sitting down to eat before they go on to other activities. My goal is to help you to take the "I don't have time" factor out of the equation.

Most of the recipes you'll find here require as little as 5 minutes of preparation and can be put together in 20 to 30 minutes max. Many of the dishes do not require cooking at all. Things like salads, smoothies, and sandwiches do not require cooking, and I will show you how to put together a meal from foods you have readily available. It's simply about putting the right ingredients together and enjoying your meal.

Following each recipe is a nutritional analysis that tells you the total calories, carbs, protein, and fat found in each recipe. There is also a percentage listed for carbs, protein, and fat that represents the percentage of these macronutrients found in the total calories. You may notice that the mass of the protein choices at each meal appears larger than the mass of carbohydrates used at each meal. However, carbohydrates are contributing to a higher percentage of the total calories of the meal. Why? Because protein choices are not solely protein. For example, chicken might be 60 percent protein and 40 percent fat. Therefore, the mass of your hand equivalent of chicken is really only 60 percent protein. On the other hand, most carbohydrate choices are primarily carbohydrate. Almost all the calories from a sweet potato or rice come from carbohydrates.

Over time, as you build your confidence in the kitchen, you will find yourself baking, stir-frying, grilling, and more as you add variety and taste to your dishes. I don't know how to flambé, I don't know how to make a proper roux, and I don't know how to make a meringue. However, I can make a smoothie in my sleep, make a variety of delicious sandwiches, and my tasty shrimp stir-fry takes only minutes to prepare.

Another benefit of following the PATH approach is that it's easy to plan meals in advance. So when you do cook, you can make enough food to provide a couple of meals—leftovers are tasty, quick, and easy. If you've got something in your fridge that's already been prepared, you're less likely to find yourself hungry without any healthy food options and succumb to ordering fast-food on your favorite food delivery app or scarfing down some empty calories.

These recipes are for quick, easy, delicious meals that will give your body everything it needs, and your appetite everything it's ever wanted. There's a little bit of something for everyone, including options for your three main meals (breakfast, lunch, and dinner) as well as snacks. I've designed these recipes so that anyone can take a few ingredients and turn them into something delicious. Bon appétit!

BREAKFAST

CEREAL AND BERRIES

Happily, there are many high-fiber cereals available. I recommend finding a brand you like that contains only a small amount of sugar and then topping your bowl with naturally sweet berries. Another great topping is crushed nuts (like hazelnuts). Five to seven crushed nuts will add crunch and lots of healthy fats.

HARLEY HACK: If you can't completely walk away from your favorite sweetened cereal, combine a high-fiber, low-sugar cereal (about 85 percent of the bowl) with a handful of sweetened cereal. If you have kids, try the trick with them to wean them away from the sugary stuff as well. Brands I like: Kashi Go, Magic Spoon, and Three Wishes.

APPLE PIE SMOOTHIE

SERVES 1

This is one of my most-requested recipes and was first introduced in my book *The Body Reset Diet.*

HARLEY HACK: Got overripe bananas? Peel and put them in a resealable bag, then freeze them for future smoothies.

5 raw almonds

1 red apple, peeled, cored, and chopped

1 small frozen banana, chopped

6 ounces nonfat plain Greek yogurt

$\frac{1}{2}$ cup nonfat milk or alternative milk of your choice

$\frac{1}{2}$ teaspoon ground cinnamon or to taste

Place the almonds in a blender or food processor and process until finely ground. Add the apple, banana, yogurt, milk, and cinnamon and blend until the desired consistency.

<u>Nutritional analysis:</u> Calories 378, carbohydrates 68 grams, protein 18 grams, fat 4 grams Carbs 72%, protein 19%, fat 9%

PB & J OATMEAL SHORT-STACK PANCAKES

SERVES 1

The classic peanut butter and jelly combination gets a makeover in these filling and protein-packed pancakes. Add any berries, either fresh or frozen, and the nut butter of your choice.

Nonstick cooking spray

1/2 cup quick oats

1/2 cup egg whites (from 4 large eggs)

1 cup fresh or thawed frozen berries

1 tablespoon peanut butter or nut butter of your choice

Lightly coat a medium nonstick skillet with cooking spray and place over medium-low heat. Combine the oats, egg whites, berries, and peanut butter in a blender or food processor, and process until well blended.

Pour about one-quarter of the mixture onto the hot skillet; use a nonstick spatula to press down on the pancake to flatten. Cook for 2 minutes, flip the pancake, and cook another minute until cooked through. Remove the pancake from the skillet and place on a plate.

Repeat making pancakes with the remaining batter, removing them from the skillet and placing them on the plate with the previously cooked pancakes. Serve immediately.

<u>Nutritional analysis:</u> Calories 440, carbohydrates 50 grams, protein 35 grams, fat 11 grams Carbs 46%, protein 31%, fat 23%

CHIA SEED PUDDING

SERVES 5

Refrigerating this miracle three-ingredient pudding overnight results in a creamy, satisfying boost for your morning. Plus, it's loaded with healthy fats!

HARLEY HACK: Because this recipe makes five servings, it's a good idea to divide the mixture into 5 mason jars and screw on the lids. That way, you'll have single-serving to-go cups for the week.

1 cup whole white chia seeds

4 cups nonfat milk or alternative milk of your choice

Dash of pure vanilla extract

Dash of pure maple syrup or sweetener of your choice

Berries for topping (optional)

Combine the chia seeds, milk, vanilla, and maple syrup in a medium bowl. Stir well, wait for 5 minutes, and stir again. Cover and refrigerate overnight. Serve topped with berries of your choice (if using).

Nutritional analysis: Calories 213, carbs 25 grams, protein 16 grams, fat 12 grams
Carbs 37%, protein 24%, fat 39%

BAKED APPLE WITH CINNAMON YOGURT

SERVES 1

Breakfast apple pie! Why not? I suggest a firm apple, like Honeycrisp or Fuji. A softer variety will melt into mush.

HARLEY HACK: Bake several apples at once and store them in the fridge for speedy weekday breakfasts. The baking time will depend on the size of your apple, so check the apple at 30 minutes and bake to your desired softness.

1 firm apple, such as
Honeycrisp or Fuji

1/2 cup nonfat plain Greek
yogurt

1/4 teaspoon ground cinnamon

5 cashews or almonds,
coarsely chopped

Preheat the oven to 350°F.

Slice off the top of the apple to create a flat surface. Using an apple corer or a paring knife, carefully cut around the core in a circle, leaving some apple at the bottom. Remove the core and seeds, creating a deep hole.

Place the apple in a small baking dish. Add about 1/2 cup water to the dish. Cover the dish with aluminum foil and bake for 30 to 40 minutes, until the apple is tender but not mushy.

Place the yogurt in a small resealable plastic bag. Add the cinnamon, seal the bag, and squeeze the bag to blend. Snip off a corner of the bag and squeeze out the yogurt into the hole of the apple. Top with nuts and serve warm.

<u>Nutritional analysis:</u> **Calories 226, carbohydrates 35 grams, protein 15 grams, fat 4 grams Carbs 59%, protein 26%, fat 15%**

SPINACH AND CHEESE OMELET

SERVES 1

Serve this colorful omelet with a side of high-fiber toast. If things go awry and the omelet isn't folding as you like, just start scrambling. It may not look as perfect, but it will taste just as delicious!

HARLEY HACK: Mash up some fresh berries to make the quickest ever homemade jam—perfect for spreading on toast.

Nonstick cooking spray

1 small red bell pepper, thinly sliced (about ½ cup)

Handful of baby spinach, chopped

⅓ cup egg whites (from 3 large eggs)

1 large egg

Salt and freshly ground black pepper

1 slice low-fat provolone or Swiss cheese (about 1 ounce)

2 slices high-fiber bread, toasted

¼ cup berries of your choice

Lightly coat a medium nonstick skillet with cooking spray and place over medium heat. Add the pepper slices and cook for 4 minutes, stirring until softened and browned in spots. Stir in the spinach and 2 tablespoons water and cook, stirring, for 2 minutes, until wilted. Remove the vegetables to a plate.

Place the skillet back over medium-low heat. Add the egg whites and whole egg, and cook for 1 minute, running a heatproof rubber spatula around the edges of the omelet to loosen it from the pan. Add the vegetables to one side of the omelet and top with the cheese. Tilt the skillet and fold half of the omelet over the vegetables. Using the spatula to lift the omelet, carefully slide the omelet onto a serving plate. Serve warm with the toast topped with the berries.

Nutritional analysis: Calories 360, carbohydrates 39 grams, protein 32 grams, fat 10 grams
Carbs 42%, protein 35%, fat 24%

CHOCOLATE-BANANA OATMEAL PANCAKES

SERVES 1

These hearty pancakes are naturally sweetened from the bananas and super satisfying from the oats. Remember to use a ripe banana for maximum sweetness.

1 cup quick oats

¼ cup nonfat milk or alternative milk of your choice

2 scoops protein powder

1 ripe banana

½ teaspoon ground cinnamon

1 teaspoon unsweetened cocoa powder

Place a nonstick skillet over medium-low heat. Combine the oats, milk, protein powder, banana, cinnamon, and cocoa in a blender or food processor, and process until well blended. Pour half of the mixture into the hot skillet; use a nonstick spatula to press down on the pancake to flatten. Cook for 2 minutes, flip the pancake, and cook another minute until cooked through. Remove the pancake from the skillet and place on a plate.

Repeat with the remaining batter. Serve immediately.

Nutritional analysis: Calories 480, carbohydrates 59 grams, protein 34 grams, fat 12 grams
Carbs 50%, protein 28%, fat 22%

BROCCOLI AND CHEESE FRITTATA WITH AVO TOAST

SERVES 1

In this healthy breakfast, I often use frozen broccoli. Because it is preserved at peak freshness, you get the maximum nutritional benefits. For easy cleanup, use an 8-inch nonstick skillet. If you have only a larger skillet, just push the mixture to one side and create a half-moon-shaped frittata. A scramble also works!

Nonstick cooking spray

1 to 2 cups chopped broccoli, fresh or frozen

Salt and freshly ground black pepper

2/3 cup egg whites (from 5 large eggs)

1 large egg

1/2 cup chopped fresh tomatoes

1 ounce shredded low-fat cheddar cheese (about 1/4 cup)

2 slices high-fiber bread, toasted

1/4 cup avocado slices

Lightly coat a small ovenproof nonstick skillet with cooking spray and place over medium heat. Stir in the broccoli and season with salt and pepper to taste. Add water to cover the broccoli, cover, and cook until the broccoli is just tender, 3 minutes.

Meanwhile, preheat the broiler.

Whisk together the egg whites and egg with the tomatoes and salt and pepper to taste in a bowl. Add the egg mixture to the skillet and stir gently until large curds form and the edges begin to set, about 30 seconds. Top with the cheese.

Transfer the skillet to the oven and broil for 2 minutes, until the eggs are puffed, golden, and just set. Serve with the toast and avocado slices.

Nutritional analysis: Calories 451, carbohydrates 41 grams, protein 41 grams, fat 15 grams Carbs 36%, protein 36%, fat 28%

BRUNCH-FOR-ONE MINI QUICHES

MAKES 4

Yes, you can treat yourself to a brunch dish at home. You deserve it.

HARLEY HACK: Whisk the ingredients together in a large glass measuring cup or medium bowl with a spout, so it's easy to pour the mixture into the muffin cups.

Nonstick cooking spray

1/4 cup diced red onion

1/2 cup jarred roasted red peppers, drained and chopped

3 small red potatoes, diced small

Handful of baby spinach, coarsely chopped

1/2 cup egg whites (from 4 large eggs)

1/2 cup nonfat milk

Salt and freshly ground black pepper

1 1/2 ounces crumbled feta cheese (about 1/4 cup)

1 high-fiber pita bread, warmed

Preheat the oven to 350°F. Lightly coat 4 muffin cups with cooking spray.

Lightly coat a medium nonstick skillet with cooking spray and place over medium-low heat. Add the onion, roasted peppers, and potatoes and cook for 5 minutes, stirring, until softened. Add the spinach and 1/4 cup water and cook for 3 minutes, stirring, until wilted.

In a large glass measuring cup or medium bowl with a spout, whisk the egg whites, milk, and salt and pepper to taste. Fold in the cooked vegetables and the cheese. Pour the mixture into the prepared muffin cups. Bake for 30 minutes, or until the mini quiches are puffed and the eggs are cooked through. Serve with the warm pita.

Nutritional analysis: Calories 457, carbohydrates 55 grams, protein 40 grams, fat 10 grams Carbs 48%, protein 33%, fat 19%

SAUSAGE, EGG, AND CHEESE BREAKFAST PASTA

SERVES 1

A classic breakfast combination takes on an energy-boosting blast with the addition of leftover pasta. Make it especially nutritious by throwing in any leftover cooked veggies you have hanging around in the refrigerator.

Nonstick cooking spray

Handful of baby spinach or baby arugula

4 ounces cooked whole wheat pasta or a gluten-free variety

1/2 cup egg whites (from 4 large eggs)

2 ounces sliced turkey pepperoni

Salt and freshly ground black pepper

1 ounce shredded low-fat cheddar cheese (about 1/4 cup)

Everything bagel seasoning (optional)

1 slice high-fiber bread, toasted

Lightly coat a medium nonstick skillet with cooking spray and place over medium-low heat. Add the spinach and cook for 1 minute, stirring. Add the cooked pasta, egg whites, and turkey pepperoni and cook for 1 minute, stirring constantly, until the eggs are cooked through.

Spoon the egg mixture onto a serving plate, season with salt and pepper to taste, and top with the cheese and everything bagel seasoning (if using). Serve with the toast.

Nutritional analysis: Calories 469, carbohydrates 50 grams, protein 40 grams, fat 9 grams Carbs 43%, protein 35%, fat 17%

FRENCH TOAST WITH QUICK BERRY SAUCE

SERVES 1

Life should include all foods, no restrictions! French toast isn't the real thing without the taste of butter and maple syrup. Just make sure to use these ingredients sparingly. Be sure to look for pure maple syrup, not the stuff labeled "pancake syrup."

HARLEY HACK: Store a loaf of high-fiber bread in the freezer for French toast. Frozen bread is really dry, meaning it absorbs the egg whites super quickly. This means you can cook the toast right away, rather than waiting for it to soak.

½ cup fresh or thawed frozen raspberries or blueberries

½ cup egg whites (from 4 large eggs)

2 tablespoons nonfat milk or milk alternative of your choice

¼ teaspoon ground cinnamon or nutmeg

½ teaspoon pure vanilla extract

Nonstick cooking spray

2 slices high-fiber bread, toasted

1 teaspoon butter

1 teaspoon pure maple syrup

Mash the berries with a fork in a small bowl until chunky. Set aside.

In a medium bowl, whisk the egg whites, milk, cinnamon, and vanilla until frothy. Add the bread slices and flip to coat.

Lightly coat a medium nonstick skillet with cooking spray and place over medium-low heat. Place the bread in the warm skillet and cook for 1 to 2 minutes per side, until golden brown and hot. Remove the toasts to a serving plate.

Reduce the heat to low. Add the mashed berries to the skillet for 15 seconds, stirring, until softened and warmed through. Top the warmed French toasts with the butter, syrup, and berry sauce.

<u>Nutritional analysis:</u> **Calories 345, carbohydrates 55 grams, protein 23 grams, fat 6 grams Carbs 60%, protein 25%, fat 15%**

VEGGIE SLAW SCRAMBLE

SERVES 1

One nutritional guideline that's easy to remember: a colorful plate is a healthy plate. This quick scramble is packed with color and reminds me of one of my favorite Japanese meals, okonomiyaki, a shredded cabbage pancake. Fiber-rich and so satisfying!

1 teaspoon olive oil

1/2 cup shredded carrots

1/2 cup shredded red cabbage

1/2 cup chopped red bell pepper

1/3 cup egg whites (from 3 large eggs)

1 large egg

Salt and freshly ground black pepper

2 slices high-fiber bread, toasted

Warm the olive oil in a medium nonstick skillet over medium heat. Add the carrots, cabbage, and bell pepper and cook for 1 minute, stirring, until slightly softened.

In a small bowl, whisk the egg whites, egg, and salt and pepper to taste. Add the mixture to the hot pan and cook for 1 minute, stirring constantly, until the eggs are cooked through. Serve immediately with the toasts.

Nutritional analysis: Calories 365, carbohydrates 45 grams, protein 29 grams, fat 12 grams Carbs 45%, protein 30%, fat 25%

APPLE CINNAMON OATMEAL

SERVES 1

For maximum fiber, leave the skin on the apple. Plus, it looks pretty atop the warm oatmeal.

HARLEY HACK: If you don't have any nuts in the house, top with a dollop of your favorite nut butter.

2 cups water

1/4 teaspoon salt

1 cup quick oats

3 scoops protein powder

1/2 teaspoon ground cinnamon

1 teaspoon butter

1 medium apple (any), chopped

1 tablespoon chopped walnuts or nut of your choice

Combine the water and salt in a small saucepan and bring to a boil over high heat. Stir in the oats and protein powder, reduce the heat to medium, and cook for 2 minutes, stirring. Remove from the heat, cover, and let stand for 3 minutes. Remove the cover and stir to incorporate any remaining liquid. Stir in the cinnamon and butter. Top with the apples and walnuts.

Nutritional analysis: Calories 421, carbohydrates 56 grams, protein 31 grams, fat 11 grams
Carbs 50%, protein 28%, fat 22%

AVOCADO MUSCLE TOAST

SERVES 1

Use your imagination to add color and crunch with your avo toast toppings, but think veggies—sliced radishes, pea shoots, shredded carrots. Or go super savory with everything bagel seasoning or crushed red pepper flakes.

2 large eggs	**Salt**
2 tablespoons avocado flesh (from 1/2 small avocado)	**1 slice high-fiber bread, toasted**

Place the eggs in a small saucepan and cover with cold water by 1 inch. Bring to a boil over high heat. Turn off the heat, cover, and let the eggs sit in the hot water for 10 minutes. Using a slotted spoon, remove the eggs from the water and place in a colander in the sink. Run cold water over the eggs to stop the cooking. Once the eggs are cool, peel them, remove the yolks, and slice the whites. Set aside the yolk to use later—in salads, deviled eggs, and so on.

Meanwhile, in a small bowl, mash the avocado with salt to taste until creamy. Spread onto the toast and top with the sliced egg whites.

Nutritional analysis: Calories 144, carbohydrates 22 grams, protein 15 grams, fat 5 grams Carbs 46%, protein 31%, fat 23%

LUNCH

TURKEY SWISS PANINI

SERVES 1

I like to make this in one of those old-fashioned sandwich grills (check out my Instagram for a video), but this satisfying sandwich also works on the stovetop.

HARLEY HACK: Because the sandwich cooks so quickly, I recommend toasting the bread first.

Nonstick cooking spray

1 teaspoon reduced-fat mayonnaise (optional)

2 slices high-fiber bread, toasted

2 thin slices turkey breast (about 2 ounces)

½ cup jarred roasted red peppers, drained and chopped

Handful of chopped baby arugula or baby spinach

2 thin slices low-fat Swiss cheese (about 1 ounce)

Lightly coat a medium nonstick skillet with cooking spray and place over medium-low heat. Spread the mayonnaise (if using) on one slice of toasted bread, then layer with turkey, roasted peppers, arugula, and cheese. Top with the remaining bread slice. Place the panini in the hot skillet and top with a smaller skillet, pressing down on the sandwich. Cook for 2 minutes, flip the panini, and cook another minute, until warmed through and the cheese is melted. Serve immediately.

Nutritional analysis: Calories 328, carbohydrates 41 grams, protein 33 grams, fat 5 grams
Carbs 48%, protein 37%, fat 14%

SKILLET GRILLED CHEESE WITH TOMATO SOUP

SERVES 1

Everyone needs a comfort food treat now and then. This childhood favorite combo is power boosted with high-fiber bread and a handful of chickpeas whipped into the tomato soup.

HARLEY HACK: Although this calls for a small amount of butter, if it's soft enough you should be able to get a nice coating on the bread.

1 cup prepared tomato soup

½ cup canned chickpeas, drained

Nonstick cooking spray

1 teaspoon softened butter

2 slices high-fiber bread, toasted

2 ounces (sliced) low-fat cheddar cheese or 1 ounce (sliced) full-fat cheddar cheese

Combine the soup and chickpeas in a blender or food processor until blended and creamy. Transfer to a small saucepan and warm over low heat.

Lightly coat a small skillet with cooking spray and place over medium-low heat. Spread the butter over one side of each bread slice. Sandwich the cheese between the unbuttered slices. Place, buttered side down, in the hot skillet and top with a smaller skillet to press down on the sandwich. Cook for 1 minute, flip the sandwich, press down, and cook another minute, until warmed through and the cheese is melted. Serve with warm soup for dipping!

Nutritional analysis: Calories 450, carbohydrates 63 grams, protein 28 grams, fat 14 grams
Carbs 51%, protein 24%, fat 25%

TUNA MELT

SERVES 1

Use this basic recipe as a quick-and-dirty (but oh so clean eating!) sandwich, then load on the veggies as desired. Celery adds crunch here, but chopped red bell pepper or tomato would add color. Feel free to substitute canned salmon if you prefer.

Nonstick cooking spray

2 ounces albacore tuna packed in water, drained

2 teaspoons reduced-fat mayonnaise

1 tablespoon fresh lemon juice or bottled lemon concentrate

2 tablespoons chopped celery

Salt and freshly ground black pepper

2 slices high-fiber bread, toasted

2 thin slices low-fat Swiss cheese (about 1 ounce) or 1 slice full-fat Swiss cheese

Lightly coat a small nonstick skillet with cooking spray and place over medium-low heat. Combine the tuna, mayonnaise, lemon juice, and celery in a medium bowl. Add salt and pepper to taste. Spoon the mixture onto one bread slice, top with the cheese, and add the remaining bread. Place the sandwich in the hot skillet and use a smaller skillet to press down on the sandwich. Cook for 2 minutes, flip the sandwich, and cook another minute, until warmed through and the cheese is melted. Serve immediately.

Nutritional analysis: Calories 338, carbohydrates 40 grams, protein 26 grams, fat 12 grams Carbs 45%, protein 28%, fat 28%

TEX-MEX STUFFED BAKED POTATO

SERVES 1

You'll have more than enough filling to fill the potato shell. For fun, use the top you slice off to scoop up the leftover filling. Think potato nacho!

HARLEY HACK: If needed, you can place the filled potato in the still-warm oven to melt the cheese. But if you time it right, combining the cooked chicken with the warm potato filling should do the trick.

1 medium russet potato

Nonstick cooking spray

3 ounces chicken tenders, sliced, or thinly sliced boneless skinless chicken breast

Salt and freshly ground black pepper

1 teaspoon taco seasoning mix

1/4 cup canned black beans, drained, or canned refried beans

1 ounce shredded low-fat cheddar cheese (about 1/4 cup)

1/4 cup mashed avocado (from about 1/4 avocado)

Chopped fresh tomatoes and sliced jalapeño or banana pepper (optional)

Preheat the oven to 400° F.

Poke the potato all over with a fork and wrap in aluminum foil. Place on a baking sheet and bake for 1 hour, until you can prick the potato easily with a fork. Unwrap the potato and carefully cut a thin slice off the top. Using a spoon, scoop out the potato flesh, place in a medium bowl, and lightly mash with a fork. Leave at least 1/4 inch of potato around the edges of the skin.

Meanwhile, lightly coat a medium nonstick skillet with cooking spray and place over medium heat. Season the chicken with salt and pepper to taste. Add the chicken to the hot skillet and cook for 2 minutes, stirring, until lightly brown. Sprinkle with the taco seasoning mix, add the beans and 2 tablespoons water, and simmer for 3 minutes, until the chicken is cooked through and the beans are warmed.

Add the chicken mixture and cheese to the potato in the bowl and stir to combine. Fill the potato skin with the mixture and top with the avocado and the tomatoes and peppers (if using). Serve immediately.

<u>Nutritional analysis:</u> **Calories 373, carbohydrates 43 grams, protein 33 grams, fat 8 grams Carbs 46%, protein 35%, fat 19%**

ANYTIME QUESADILLA

SERVES 1

This recipe calls for cooked chicken or shrimp, but I also recommend stocking up on canned protein sources like chicken, salmon, and tuna.

HARLEY HACK: There's no need to measure out the greens here; just add a big handful to the skillet. Remember that greens like arugula and spinach cook down *a lot*.

Nonstick cooking spray

2 high-fiber tortillas

2 ounces cooked chicken breast or cooked shrimp, chopped

1/2 cup jarred roasted red peppers, drained and chopped

2 slices fresh tomato or 2 tablespoons prepared marinara sauce

1 ounce shredded part-skim mozzarella cheese (about 1/4 cup)

Handful of baby arugula or baby spinach

Lightly coat a medium nonstick skillet with cooking spray and place over medium-low heat. Top one tortilla with the chicken, peppers, tomato, cheese, and arugula. Top with the remaining tortilla. Place the quesadilla in the hot skillet. Cook for 1 minute until lightly browned, flip the quesadilla, and cook another minute until warmed through and the cheese is melted. Serve immediately.

Nutritional analysis: Calories 422, carbohydrates 49 grams, protein 36 grams, fat 15 grams
Carbs 46%, protein 34%, fat 30%

TURKEY REUBEN ON RYE

SERVES 1

A deli classic made healthier by using lean turkey and low-fat cheese. However, you can absolutely add a splash of the traditional Thousand Island dressing.

HARLEY HACK: Got a sandwich press? Pull it out for a warm, cheesy sandwich.

Nonstick cooking spray

2 teaspoons reduced-fat Thousand Island dressing

2 slices thin rye bread or high-fiber bread

3 ounces sliced turkey breast

1 ounce slice of low-fat Swiss cheese

1/4 cup prepared sauerkraut or oil-based coleslaw

Lightly coat a medium nonstick skillet with cooking spray and place over medium-low heat. Spread the dressing on one slice of bread. Layer on the turkey, cheese, and sauerkraut and top with the remaining bread slice. Place the sandwich in the hot skillet and top with a smaller skillet, pressing down on the sandwich. Cook for 2 minutes, flip the sandwich, and cook another minute, until warmed through and the cheese is melted. Serve immediately.

Nutritional analysis: Calories 308, carbohydrates 36 grams, protein 28 grams, fat 5 grams Carbs 48%, protein 37%, fat 15%

CLASSIC CHOPPED SALAD WITH HOMEMADE CROUTONS

SERVES 1

Don't let the list of ingredients dissuade you from making this bright and crisp salad. Many ingredients, tons of flavor, very little work.

HARLEY HACK: Got leftover bread that's getting a little stale? Dice those slices and bake in a toaster oven or low oven until lightly brown and crisp. Croutons, yes!

1 slice high-fiber bread

1 teaspoon olive oil

1 teaspoon balsamic vinegar

3 cups chopped romaine lettuce

10 cherry tomatoes, halved

2 ounces sliced turkey breast (about 2 thin slices), diced

1/2 cup chopped cucumber (about 1/2 small cucumber)

1/2 cup diced green or red bell pepper

1/2 cup canned chickpeas, drained

1 ounce diced or shredded part-skim mozzarella cheese (about 1/4 cup)

Toast the bread and cut it into cubes. Set aside.

Combine the oil and vinegar in a medium serving bowl and whisk until blended. Add the romaine, tomatoes, turkey, cucumber, bell pepper, chickpeas, and cheese, and toss to coat. Top with the croutons and serve immediately.

Nutritional analysis: Calories 405, carbohydrates 45 grams, protein 32 grams, fat 10 grams Carbs 46%, protein 32%, fat 23%

FIVE-MINUTE WRAP

SERVES 1

Loaded with colorful vegetables and protein-packed, this quick lunch wrap will power you through even the hardest of days. Plant-based folks may replace the turkey with tofu or additional chickpeas. Feel free to swap in your veggies of choice.

- 1/4 cup avocado flesh (from about 1/4 avocado)
- 1 teaspoon fresh lemon juice or bottled lemon concentrate
- Salt
- 1 large high-fiber tortilla

- 3 ounces sliced turkey breast
- 1/2 cup shredded carrot
- 1/2 cup shredded red cabbage
- 1/4 cup pea shoots or alfalfa sprouts

Coarsely mash the avocado, lemon juice, and salt to taste with a fork in a small bowl. Spread the mixture over the tortilla. Top with the turkey, carrot, cabbage, and pea shoots. Roll up the wrap, cut it in half, and serve immediately.

Nutritional analysis: Calories 300, carbohydrates 35 grams, protein 25 grams, fat 8 grams Carbs 46%, protein 32%, fat 24%

SWEET POTATO AND BLACK BEAN BURRITO

SERVES 1

Sweet potatoes and black beans are a superfood combination—plant-based protein, fiber, and tons of antioxidants. Remember to eat those fiber-rich sweet potato skins.

HARLEY HACK: Just a spoonful of fresh lime juice turns plain yogurt into a lush, lime-cream topping.

Nonstick cooking spray

$1/4$ cup diced red onion

1 garlic clove, minced

1 cup shredded sweet potato (from about $1/2$ medium potato)

$1/2$ cup canned black beans, drained, or canned refried beans

$1/2$ teaspoon taco seasoning mix

Salt and freshly ground black pepper

1 ounce shredded low-fat cheddar cheese (about $1/4$ cup)

2 tablespoons nonfat plain Greek yogurt

1 tablespoon fresh lime juice or bottled lime concentrate

1 large high-fiber tortilla, warmed

Chopped iceberg or romaine lettuce, sliced jalapeño or banana pepper, or chopped fresh cilantro (optional)

Lightly coat a medium nonstick skillet with cooking spray and place over medium-low heat. Add the red onion and garlic and cook for 2 minutes, stirring, until softened. Add the sweet potatoes, beans, taco seasoning mix, and salt and pepper to taste. Cover and cook for 6 to 8 minutes, stirring frequently and adding a splash of water to make sure it's not sticking. When the sweet potato is tender, remove from the heat and stir in the cheese.

Meanwhile, combine the yogurt and lime juice in a small bowl.

Spread the tortilla with the sweet potato mixture and top with the lettuce, sliced peppers, or cilantro (if using), and the lime cream. Roll up and serve immediately.

<u>Nutritional analysis:</u> Calories 416, carbohydrates 70 grams, protein 26 grams, fat 11 grams
Carbs 58%, protein 22%, fat 20%

MARINARA PIZZA POCKET

SERVES 1

If you have a sandwich press, use it, as it creates a toasty pocket filled with sauce and melty cheese. A nonstick skillet works as well, but keep an eye on the sandwich. With so little fat in the pan, the bread burns quickly. You might need to turn down the heat to ensure the cheese melts in such a quick cooking time.

HARLEY HACK: An easy time-saver—look for a marinara sauce with added flavors, like basil or garlic. Just make sure the sauce doesn't also include lots of sugar.

Nonstick cooking spray

2 tablespoons prepared marinara sauce

2 slices high-fiber bread, toasted

Handful of baby spinach

1 ounce shredded part-skim mozzarella cheese (about ¼ cup)

Crushed red pepper flakes (optional)

Lightly coat a medium nonstick skillet with cooking spray and place over medium-low heat. Spread the marinara sauce on a slice of toasted bread, then layer on the spinach, cheese, and red pepper flakes (if using). Top with the remaining bread slice. Place the sandwich in the hot skillet and top with a smaller skillet to press down on the sandwich. Cook for 2 minutes, flip the sandwich, and cook another minute, until warmed through and the cheese is melted. Serve immediately.

Nutritional analysis: Calories 290, carbohydrates 45 grams, protein 18 grams, fat 10 grams
Carbs 53%, protein 22%, fat 25%

WEEKDAY TURKEY CHILI

SERVES 2

Use this basic recipe to make it your own; substitute a different protein or another bean. Ground chicken would be great here, too. If you've got garnishes in the fridge, shower your chili with chopped herbs or sliced jalapeño. Also, look for tomato sauce that is boosted with additional flavors like garlic or is fire-roasted.

HARLEY HACK: Because it's annoying to use only part of a can of beans, this recipe serves two. It will keep for several days in the fridge.

Nonstick cooking spray

6 ounces lean ground turkey

¼ cup chopped onion

2 garlic cloves, minced

1 tablespoon chili powder

Salt and freshly ground black pepper

1 cup tomato sauce or prepared marinara sauce

1 can (15 ounces) red kidney beans, drained

Nonfat plain Greek yogurt, sliced jalapeño pepper, or chopped fresh cilantro (optional)

Whole wheat roll, high-fiber bread, or warmed cooked rice

Lightly coat a medium saucepan with nonstick cooking spray and place over medium-low heat. Add the turkey, onion, garlic, chili powder, and salt and pepper to taste. Cook for 7 minutes, stirring, until the meat is lightly browned and no longer pink. Add the tomato sauce and beans, reduce the heat to low, and cook for 5 minutes, stirring often and if the mixture seems dry adding water a tablespoon at a time, until the desired consistency.

Ladle the chili into a serving bowl and top with yogurt, jalapeño, or cilantro (if using). Serve with the bread or warmed rice.

Nutritional analysis: Calories 483, carbohydrates 66 grams, protein 34 grams, fat 12 grams
Carbs 52%, protein 21%, fat 21%

SUPER-STUFFED BAKED SWEET POTATO

SERVES 1

Pairing sweet potato and hummus is a wonderful flavor combination, not to mention a powerhouse blend of fiber and protein. Just remember to eat every bite of the sweet potato skin!

1 medium sweet potato

Nonstick cooking spray

3 ounces fresh or frozen shrimp, halved, or canned shrimp

Salt and freshly ground black pepper

2 big handfuls of baby spinach

1 ounce crumbled low-fat feta cheese (about ¼ cup)

2 tablespoons prepared hummus or Homemade Hummus (page 190)

1 teaspoon fresh lime or lemon juice or bottled lime or lemon concentrate

Preheat the oven to 400°F.

Poke the sweet potato with a fork and wrap it in aluminum foil. Place on a baking sheet and bake for 1 hour, until you can prick the sweet potato easily with a fork. Unwrap the sweet potato and carefully cut a thin slice off the top. Using a spoon, scoop out the flesh, place it in a medium bowl, and lightly mash it with a fork. Leave at least ¼ inch of sweet potato around the edges. Set aside.

Meanwhile, lightly coat a medium nonstick skillet with cooking spray and place over medium heat. Season the shrimp with salt and pepper to taste. Add to the hot skillet and cook for 3 minutes, stirring and flipping the shrimp halfway through, until lightly golden. Add the spinach and cook for 2 minutes more, stirring, until wilted.

Add the shrimp mixture and cheese to the reserved warm sweet potato and stir to combine. Scoop the shrimp and sweet potato mixture into the sweet potato skin. Top with the hummus, sprinkle with the lime juice, and serve immediately.

Nutritional analysis: Calories 375, carbohydrates 62 grams, protein 30 grams, fat 17 grams Carbs 55%, protein 28%, fat 17%

SPRINGTIME CHOPPED SALAD

SERVES 1

This fresh, bright, no-cook salad makes a perfect quick lunch (or dinner). Use the meat from a rotisserie chicken or open a tin of canned chicken. Use a vegetable peeler to shave the asparagus spears; no need to cook!

HARLEY HACK: Feel free to substitute your favorite veggies here. Check out the salad bar at your grocery store and select a variety of options for salads for the week.

- 2 teaspoons olive oil
- 2 teaspoons fresh lemon juice or bottled lemon concentrate
- 3 cups chopped romaine lettuce
- 4 asparagus spears, shaved
- ½ cup shredded carrot
- ½ cup pea shoots or alfalfa sprouts
- 3 ounces cooked chicken breast, diced
- 1 high-fiber pita bread, warmed if desired

Combine the oil and lemon juice in a medium serving bowl and whisk until blended. Add the romaine, asparagus, carrot, pea shoots, and chicken, and toss to coat with the dressing. Serve with the pita.

Nutritional analysis: Calories 405, carbohydrates 45 grams, protein 32 grams, fat 10 grams Carbs 46%, protein 32%, fat 23%

SALMON CAESAR SALAD BURRITO

SERVES 1

Canned salmon is a busy cook's dream: not only is it super convenient, it also can hang out in your pantry ready to make the quickest of meals. More good news: it's high in protein and healthy fats. Most people prefer the smooth texture of the boneless skinless type, but those that include the bones provide more calcium. Just add a creamy lemon dressing, some juicy tomatoes, and wrap it up in a high-fiber tortilla. If you are really in a hurry, you can substitute prepared Caesar dressing for the yogurt-lemon dressing, but make sure it's a low-sugar, reduced-fat dressing.

HARLEY HACK: Not all tortillas are alike; take a close look at the nutritional facts to make sure you select a high-fiber, low-sugar brand.

- 3 ounces canned salmon packed in water
- 2 tablespoons nonfat plain Greek yogurt
- 1 teaspoon reduced-fat mayonnaise (optional)
- 1 teaspoon fresh lemon juice or bottled lemon concentrate
- 1 small garlic clove, minced (optional)
- Salt and freshly ground black pepper
- 1 large high-fiber tortilla
- 1 tablespoon grated Parmesan cheese
- ¼ cup chopped fresh tomato
- 1 cup shredded romaine lettuce

Combine the salmon, yogurt, mayonnaise (if using), lemon juice, garlic (if using), and salt and pepper to taste in a medium bowl. Stir and spoon the mixture onto the tortilla. Top with the cheese, tomato, and lettuce. Roll up and serve immediately.

<u>Nutritional analysis:</u> Calories 360, carbohydrates 40 grams, protein 31 grams, fat 11 grams Carbs 43%, protein 32%, fat 25%

DINNER

POACHED SALMON WITH DILL SAUCE

SERVES 1

This dish looks so elegant, but it's so easy! Bonus: poached salmon is delicious served hot or cold, so go ahead and double the quantity of fish and refrigerate half for a quick cold lunch.

HARLEY HACK: Starting the salmon cooking in cold water and then slowly heating it prevents the exterior from seizing up and becoming tough.

- **2 tablespoons fresh lemon juice or bottled lemon concentrate**
- **2 sprigs fresh dill or flat-leaf parsley, plus 1 tablespoon, chopped**
- **Salt and freshly ground black pepper**
- **4 ounces boneless skinless salmon fillet**

- **Nonstick cooking spray**
- **3 handfuls of baby spinach**
- **¼ cup nonfat plain Greek yogurt**
- **¼ teaspoon Dijon mustard**
- **1 cup cooked grain, such as quinoa, farro, or bulgur, warmed, or 1 slice high-fiber bread**

Combine 2 cups cold water, 1 tablespoon of the lemon juice, the dill sprigs, and a pinch of salt in a medium saucepan. Add the salmon and more water if needed to cover the fish. Bring to a simmer over medium-low heat. Keep the poaching liquid to a low simmer; do not let the water boil. Cook for 10 to 15 minutes, or until cooked through. (If you have a thermometer, cook until it registers 115°F.) Remove from the heat, transfer to a serving plate, and discard the poaching liquid.

Lightly coat the same saucepan with cooking spray and place over medium-low heat. Add the spinach and cook for 4 minutes, stirring, until wilted.

In a small bowl, combine the yogurt, mustard, chopped dill, and the remaining 1 tablespoon lemon juice. Season with salt and pepper to taste.

Place the salmon on a serving plate, top with the yogurt sauce, and serve with the spinach and a warmed grain or bread.

Nutritional analysis: Calories 393, carbohydrates 49 grams, protein 36 grams, fat 7 grams
Carbs 50%, protein 35%, fat 16%

THAI FUSION TACO

SERVES 1

A five-minute dinner? Sign me up! Especially when it's a bright and crunchy no-cook taco.

HARLEY HACK: Depending on the brand, and your desires, you may wish to toast your tortillas in a warm skillet or toaster oven.

2 teaspoons regular peanut butter or nut butter of your choice

2 teaspoons reduced-sodium soy sauce

1 teaspoon lime chili sauce

1 teaspoon fresh lime juice or bottled lime concentrate, plus more for garnish

3 ounces shredded cooked chicken breast

2 high-fiber tortillas, lightly toasted

½ cup shredded cabbage and carrot blend

Combine the peanut butter, soy sauce, lime chili sauce, and lime juice in a medium bowl and whisk together. Add 1 to 2 tablespoons water to achieve the consistency of heavy cream. Fold in the shredded chicken until combined.

Create tacos by filling each tortilla with chicken mixture and top with shredded cabbage and carrot blend and a splash of lime. Serve immediately.

<u>Nutritional analysis:</u> Calories 375, carbohydrates 48 grams, protein 44 grams, fat 12 grams Carbs 42%, protein 35%, fat 23%

SIMPLE CHICKEN STIR-FRY

SERVES 1

Once you get the basic instructions for stir-fry down, you can experiment with whatever protein source or veggies you have in your fridge or freezer. Frozen shrimp are a great option.

Note: We call for 2 cups of veggies here, but if you want more, just add more (and use a bigger skillet). The cooking time will vary according to the protein and vegetables used.

HARLEY HACK: We always have leftover rice after ordering Chinese, so a stir-fry is a great next-night dinner plan. But you can also buy frozen cooked rice to have on hand.

2 teaspoons olive oil

4 ounces chicken tenders or thinly sliced boneless skinless chicken breast

Salt and freshly ground black pepper

2 cups frozen mixed vegetables or chopped vegetables of your choice

¼ cup reduced-sodium chicken broth or water

2 teaspoons reduced-sodium soy sauce

1 teaspoon chili garlic sauce

1 cup cooked rice, warmed

Place 1 teaspoon of the oil in a large nonstick skillet and warm over medium to medium-high heat. Season the chicken with salt and pepper to taste. Add to the skillet and stir-fry for 3 minutes, until lightly browned but not cooked through. Remove to a plate. Add the remaining 1 teaspoon oil to the hot skillet. Stir in the vegetables and 2 tablespoons water and cook for 3 to 5 minutes, stirring, until cooked through. Return the chicken to the skillet, add the soy sauce and chili sauce, and stir until the mixture is coated with sauce and hot. Serve over the warm rice.

Nutritional analysis: Calories 438, carbohydrates 52 grams, protein 30 grams, fat 11 grams
Carbs 50%, protein 28%, fat 22%

BOUILLABAISSE

SERVES 1

My take on bouillabaisse, a classic French fish stew that traditionally features several different types of seafood and shellfish, fennel, saffron, and white wine. I've pared down the recipe to make it with more easily available ingredients, and a super-quick cooking time.

HARLEY HACK: Make sure the cooking broth completely covers the shrimp. Add broth or water if it doesn't.

1 teaspoon olive oil

¼ cup diced onion

¼ cup diced celery

¼ cup diced carrot

2 small red potatoes, diced (about ½ cup)

Salt and freshly ground black pepper

1 garlic clove, minced

1 cup prepared marinara sauce or tomato sauce

½ cup fish broth, vegetable broth, or water

4 ounces fresh or frozen large shrimp (about 8 pieces)

1 slice high-fiber bread, toasted

Place the oil in a medium saucepan and warm over medium-low heat. Add the onion, celery, carrot, and potatoes, and season with salt and pepper to taste. Cook for 7 minutes, stirring occasionally. Add the garlic, marinara sauce, and broth. Bring to a simmer and cook for 5 minutes, stirring, until thickened. Add the shrimp and cook for 5 more minutes, until the shrimp are cooked through and the potatoes are tender. Serve immediately with the toast.

<u>Nutritional analysis:</u> **Calories 440, carbohydrates 64 grams, protein 26 grams, fat 9 grams Carbs 59%, protein 23%, fat 18%**

RATATOUILLE WITH GRILLED SHRIMP

SERVES 1

Basil pesto is the traditional herb to add to this savory stew, but feel free to leave it out, or substitute something else (flat-leaf parsley! hot sauce!). If you've got dried Italian seasoning, season the shrimp with it.

HARLEY HACK: Shrimp cook super fast, so keep an eye on them. You can absolutely use frozen shrimp here. You can even grill them without waiting for them to thaw. You'll just need to cook them a little longer.

1/2 cup chopped eggplant

1/2 cup chopped zucchini

1/2 cup chopped red bell pepper

1/2 cup chopped red onion

1 cup prepared marinara sauce or tomato sauce

Salt and freshly ground black pepper

Nonstick cooking spray

4 ounces fresh or frozen large shrimp (about 8 pieces)

1 tablespoon prepared basil pesto

1 slice high-fiber bread or pita bread

Combine the eggplant, zucchini, bell pepper, red onion, marinara sauce, and 1/2 cup water in a medium saucepan. Season with salt and pepper to taste and bring to a simmer over medium heat. Reduce the heat to low, cover, and simmer for 1 hour, stirring occasionally, until the vegetables are tender. (Add water as needed to just cover the vegetables as they cook.)

Meanwhile, preheat a grill or lightly coat a grill pan with cooking spray and place over medium-high heat. Season the shrimp with salt and pepper to taste, add to the grill or grill pan, and cook for 3 minutes on each side, until pink.

Spoon the ratatouille into a shallow bowl and top with the pesto. Serve with the shrimp and bread to scoop up the stew.

<u>Nutritional analysis:</u> Calories 425, carbohydrates 65 grams, protein 28 grams, fat 8 grams Carbs 58%, protein 25%, fat 16%

VEGGIE FRIED RICE

SERVES 1

Fried rice is a wonderful way to use leftover rice, but if you don't have any, you can now find frozen cooked rice in many markets. Just remember to get your pan superhot to create those delicious crusty bits. If you have a wok, use it—otherwise a heavy nonstick pan will suffice.

HARLEY HACK: Use any veggie you prefer in this recipe or purchase a bag of frozen mixed veggies to have on hand for this quick meal. Because veggies add so few calories, feel free to add as much as you like!

Nonstick cooking spray

1 cup cooked rice

1 teaspoon olive oil

1½ cups chopped fresh or frozen broccoli

½ cup frozen or fresh edamame

1 teaspoon reduced-sodium soy sauce

1 teaspoon chili garlic sauce or dark sesame oil

Salt and freshly ground black pepper

⅓ cup egg whites (from 3 large eggs)

1 tablespoon chopped roasted peanuts (salted or unsalted)

Lightly coat a large heavy nonstick skillet with cooking spray and place over medium-high heat. Add the rice to the skillet and spread it out, pressing it up the sides, leaving enough space in the middle of the pan for the veggies. Add the oil to the space. Add the broccoli and edamame to the oil and cook for 2 minutes, stirring gently, then fold the vegetables into the rice to combine. Fold in the soy sauce and chili sauce until the ingredients are coated. Season with salt and pepper to taste. Reduce the heat to medium and push the rice mixture to one side of the skillet. Add the egg whites to the bare side of the skillet. Use a spatula to scramble the egg whites, breaking them up into small bits. Blend the egg whites and rice and serve immediately, topped with the peanuts.

Nutritional analysis: Calories 418, carbohydrates 48 grams, protein 25 grams, fat 12 grams Carbs 48%, protein 25%, fat 27%

GREEK CHICKEN SOUVLAKI PLATTER

SERVES 1

This is a meal for when you have a little more time and want to mix up your usual dinner fare. Souvlaki is a casual Greek dish redolent with Mediterranean flavors of garlic and oregano. After quickly grilling the chicken, slide the meat onto a warmed pita and slather it with tzatziki and fresh tomato slices.

HARLEY HACK: No cooked potatoes in the house? Substitute bell peppers or thick onion slices to add to your skewer.

CHICKEN SOUVLAKI

1 teaspoon olive oil

1 teaspoon fresh lemon juice or bottled lemon concentrate

1/2 teaspoon dried oregano

1 small garlic clove, minced

Salt and freshly ground black pepper

Nonstick cooking spray

3 ounces chicken tenders (2–3 tenders), or thin sliced boneless skinless chicken breasts

3 ounces cooked red potatoes

TZATZIKI

1/2 cup nonfat plain Greek yogurt

1/2 cup shredded or diced cucumber

1 teaspoon fresh lemon juice or bottled lemon concentrate

Garlic salt or 1 small garlic clove, minced

TO SERVE

1 high-fiber pita bread, warmed

Sliced tomatoes

Combine the oil, lemon juice, oregano, garlic, and salt and pepper to taste in a medium bowl and stir together. Add the chicken and stir to coat. Cover and refrigerate for at least 10 minutes or overnight.

Meanwhile, in a small bowl, combine the yogurt, cucumber, lemon juice, and garlic salt and stir together.

Preheat a grill or grill pan to medium heat and lightly coat with cooking spray.

Thread the chicken and potatoes onto wooden or metal skewers. Grill the skewers for 8 minutes, turning often, until the chicken is cooked through.

Create a platter of skewers, tzatziki, pita, and tomatoes. Slide the chicken and potatoes onto the pita, top with the tzatziki and tomatoes, and enjoy.

<u>Nutritional analysis:</u> **Calories 450, carbohydrates 55 grams, protein 48 grams, fat 10 grams Carbs 45%, protein 37%, fat 18%**

SPEEDY AND SPICY PASTA ARRABBIATA

SERVES 1

The word *arrabbiata* means "angry" in Italian—referring here to the spiciness of the sauce. Make this as bold as you dare by adding more red pepper flakes and garlic. If you are a garlic lover, buy a jar of peeled garlic and store it in your fridge to save time. Or purchase a prepared marinara sauce with added garlic.

HARLEY HACK: Be sure to check the ingredient list of your marinara sauce. These sauces can be a time-saving lifesaver for dinner prep, but some varieties are loaded with sugar.

- 4 ounces whole wheat pasta or a gluten-free variety
- 1 teaspoon olive oil
- 2 big handfuls of baby spinach, chopped
- 3/4 cup prepared marinara sauce or tomato sauce
- 2 garlic cloves, chopped
- 1/4 cup egg whites (from 2 large eggs)
- Crushed red pepper flakes
- 2 tablespoons grated Parmesan cheese

Cook the pasta in a medium saucepan according to the package directions. Drain.

Meanwhile, place the oil in a medium nonstick skillet and warm over medium-low heat. Add the spinach and cook for 2 minutes, stirring, until wilted. Add the marinara sauce, garlic, egg whites, and red pepper flakes to taste and stir to combine, smashing the egg whites against the side of the skillet to break up the cooked bits.

Combine the hot pasta and sauce in a serving bowl, toss, and top with the cheese. Serve immediately.

<u>Nutritional analysis:</u> Calories 434, carbohydrates 52 grams, protein 30 grams, fat 10 grams
Carbs 50%, protein 28%, fat 22%

CHICKEN PARMESAN WITH ROASTED VEGGIES

SERVES 1

This is a full meal! Although it's called chicken Parm, I often choose to use part-skim mozzarella because of the cheesy goodness. Using tenders rather than chicken breasts means there's no need to get out a mallet to pound the meat thin. Just press down with your (covered) palm on each tender to flatten to about 1/4-inch thickness.

The roasting time for the veggies is an estimate here—yours will depend on the type you choose and your desired doneness.

HARLEY HACK: Save time and add flavor by using Italian seasoned breadcrumbs.

- 1 cup chopped fresh or thawed frozen vegetables of your choice
- Salt and freshly ground black pepper
- 4 ounces chicken tenders (about 3), flattened to about 1/4-inch thickness
- 2 egg whites, whisked
- 1/4 cup panko or other breadcrumbs
- 1/4 teaspoon dried thyme
- 1/4 teaspoon dried oregano
- Nonstick cooking spray
- 1/2 cup marinara sauce or tomato sauce
- 1 ounce shredded part-skim mozzarella or Parmesan cheese (about 1/4 cup)
- 1 high-fiber roll or 1/2 whole wheat hamburger bun, warmed

Preheat the oven to 400°F.

Toss the veggies with salt and pepper to taste in a medium bowl. Spread out onto a baking sheet and place in oven and roast for 15 minutes, or until cooked through and lightly browned. Remove from oven and set aside.

Meanwhile, season the chicken tenders with salt and pepper to taste. Create two dipping bowls: one with whisked egg whites and one with a combination of panko, thyme, and oregano. Dip the chicken in the egg whites, letting any excess drip off, then dredge in the panko mixture, turning to coat both sides.

Lightly coat a medium nonstick skillet with cooking spray and place over medium-low heat. Cook the tenders for 3 minutes per side, until golden brown and cooked through. Transfer to an aluminum-foil-lined baking sheet. Spoon the marinara sauce over the centers of each tender, leaving the sides bare. Sprinkle with the cheese. Place in the oven and bake for 3 minutes, until the cheese melts. Serve the tenders with the warmed bun and veggies.

Nutritional analysis: Calories 500, carbohydrates 58 grams, protein 43 grams, fat 10 grams Carbs 48%, protein 35%, fat 18%

HONEY-MUSTARD TURKEY BURGER WITH OVEN-ROASTED SWEET POTATO FRIES

SERVES 1

Burger and fries hit the spot . . . especially when you can enjoy the meal knowing you are feeding your body with protein, fiber, and healthy carbs. Look for 99% lean ground turkey.

HARLEY HACK: Preheating the baking sheet in the oven makes for crispier fries and a quicker cooking time.

SWEET POTATOES

- 1 small sweet potato, sliced into ¼-inch-thick matchsticks
- Nonstick cooking spray
- Salt and freshly ground black pepper

TURKEY BURGER

- 4 ounces lean ground turkey
- 1 teaspoon Dijon or brown mustard
- 1 teaspoon Worcestershire sauce
- 1 teaspoon honey
- ¼ teaspoon garlic powder
- Salt and freshly ground black pepper
- ½ whole wheat hamburger bun
- Tomato slices, lettuce leaves, or pickles for garnish (optional)

Place a baking sheet in the oven and preheat the oven to 425°F.

Combine the sweet potato slices, cooking spray, and salt and pepper to taste in a medium bowl and toss together. Slide the slices onto the hot baking sheet and roast in the oven for 20 minutes, stirring occasionally, until crisp and cooked through.

In the same medium bowl, use your hands to combine the turkey, mustard, Worcestershire, honey, garlic powder, and salt and pepper to taste. Form the mixture into a ¾-inch-thick patty.

Lightly coat a small nonstick skillet with cooking spray and place over medium heat. Add the burger, cook for 2 minutes, flip the burger, and cook for 2 more minutes. Cover the pan and cook for 4 more minutes, until cooked through and lightly browned but still juicy. Place the burger on the bun half and garnish with tomatoes, lettuce, or pickle (if using). Serve immediately with the sweet potatoes.

Nutritional analysis: Calories 389, carbohydrates 45 grams, protein 27 grams, fat 10 grams
Carbs 48%, protein 28%, fat 24%

SHRIMP SKEWERS WITH PARMESAN AND PEA FUSILLI

SERVES 1

There are so many pasta choices at the markets now: bean-based, quinoa, whole grain, to name but a few. This means you can add solid amounts of protein and fiber and still enjoy pasta. This delicious meal includes ingredients you might not think would fit into your diet. . . . Butter! Cheese! Peas! Remember, no food is off-limits!

4 ounces whole wheat pasta or a gluten-free variety

Nonstick cooking spray

4 ounces fresh or frozen large shrimp (about 8 pieces)

Salt and freshly ground black pepper

2 handfuls of baby arugula or baby spinach

⅓ cup frozen peas (no need to thaw)

1 teaspoon butter

2 tablespoons grated Parmesan cheese

Cook the pasta in a medium saucepan according to the package directions.

Preheat a grill or lightly coat a grill pan or nonstick skillet with cooking spray and place over medium-high heat. Thread the shrimp onto wooden or metal skewers and season with salt and pepper to taste. Place the skewers on the grill or skillet and cook for 3 minutes per side.

Meanwhile, place the arugula and peas in a large colander set in the sink. When the pasta is cooked according to your preference, slowly drain the boiling water and pasta into the colander. Shake the colander to get rid of as much water as possible. Pour the colander contents into the same saucepan and set over medium heat. Add the butter and cook for 5 minutes, stirring, until the peas are warmed through and the arugula is wilted. Transfer to a serving bowl, garnish with the cheese, and arrange the shrimp skewers on top. Serve immediately.

Nutritional analysis: Calories 390, carbohydrates 48 grams, protein 29 grams, fat 10 grams Carbs 50%, protein 29%, fat 21%

CHICKEN PAILLARD ON A BED OF ARUGULA AND CHERRY TOMATOES

SERVES 1

I've increased the fiber in the salad by chopping brussels sprouts and adding them to the arugula. No—they don't need to be cooked. If you don't have any brussels sprouts, add some sliced cabbage or extra arugula.

HARLEY HACK: To make quick-cooking thin chicken pieces, place the chicken inside a gallon-size ziplock bag and seal the bag, pressing out as much air as possible. Pound with the flat side of a meat mallet, a rolling pin, or a small skillet to an even 1/4-inch thickness. Remember to discard the marinade, as it has been in contact with raw chicken.

- **1 teaspoon olive oil**
- **4 teaspoons fresh lemon juice or bottled lemon concentrate**
- **1/4 teaspoon garlic powder**
- **Salt and freshly ground black pepper**
- **4 ounces boneless skinless chicken breast, pounded to 1/4-inch thickness**

- **2 tablespoons flour, any variety**
- **Nonstick cooking spray**
- **3 cups baby arugula**
- **1 cup finely chopped brussels sprouts (optional)**
- **1/2 cup cherry tomatoes, halved**
- **1 slice high-fiber bread, warmed**

Combine the oil, 2 teaspoons of the lemon juice, the garlic powder, and salt and pepper to taste in a medium bowl. Add the chicken and turn to coat. Let marinate for 10 minutes. Place the flour and salt and pepper to taste in another medium bowl. Using a fork, add the marinated chicken to the bowl and turn to coat with the flour mixture.

Lightly coat a medium nonstick skillet with cooking spray and place over medium heat. Add the chicken and cook for 2 or 3 minutes per side, until cooked through.

Pile the arugula and chopped brussels sprouts (if using) on a serving plate, and toss with the remaining 2 teaspoons lemon juice. Top with the chicken, garnish with the cherry tomatoes, and serve with the warm bread.

Nutritional analysis: Calories 382, carbohydrates 44 grams, protein 30 grams, fat 10 grams Carbs 46%, protein 31%, fat 23%

BIBIMBAP

SERVES 1

Our take on this bright and fresh Korean classic is infinitely customizable; make it as simple or as elaborate as you like. Yes, this ingredient list is long, but the dish is ready in 5 minutes!

HARLEY HACK: Sesame seeds are optional, but just a teaspoon adds a blast of flavor, not to mention healthy fat.

Nonstick cooking spray

4 ounces fresh or frozen large shrimp (about 8 pieces)

1 teaspoon reduced-sodium soy sauce

1/2 teaspoon chili lime sauce

Salt and freshly ground black pepper

1/2 cup prepared kimchi

1 large egg

1/2 cup shredded carrot

1/2 cup sliced cucumber

1/2 cup fresh or frozen thawed edamame

3/4 cup cooked rice or grain of your choice, warmed

1 teaspoon sesame seeds (optional)

Lightly coat a medium nonstick skillet with cooking spray and place over medium heat. Combine the shrimp, soy sauce, and chili lime sauce in a small bowl. Add to the hot skillet and cook for 1 minute. Flip the shrimp and cook for 2 more minutes, or until no longer pink. Transfer to a serving bowl.

Coat the skillet again with cooking spray and place over medium-low heat. Add the kimchi to one side of the skillet. Crack the egg onto the empty side of the skillet and cook for 30 seconds. Cover the pan and cook for 3 more minutes, until the yolk is set.

Add the warmed rice to the bowl with the shrimp. Top with the kimchi, carrot, cucumber, and edamame. Place the cooked egg on top, sprinkle with sesame seeds (if using), and serve.

Nutritional analysis: Calories 445, carbohydrates 54 grams, protein 33 grams, fat 11 grams Carbs 48%, protein 30%, fat 22%

EASY CHICKEN TIKKA MASALA

SERVES 1

This flavorful meal contains more ingredients than most of my recipes, but I promise it's worth it. To save time, double the recipe so you have dinner ready to go for tomorrow night.

HARLEY HACK: Coarsely chop the cauliflower florets into small pieces so that they cook through in the short cooking time.

- 6 ounces nonfat plain Greek yogurt
- 1/4 teaspoon ground cumin
- 1/4 teaspoon ground turmeric
- 1 teaspoon fresh lime juice or bottled lime concentrate
- 4 ounces boneless skinless chicken breast, cut into 1-inch cubes
- Nonstick cooking spray

- 1/2 cup diced onion
- 1 to 2 cups cauliflower florets
- 1 teaspoon chopped fresh ginger
- 1/2 cup tomato sauce or prepared marinara sauce
- Salt and freshly ground black pepper
- 3/4 cup cooked rice, warmed

Preheat the broiler.

Combine 1/3 cup of the yogurt, the cumin, turmeric, and lime juice in a medium bowl and stir until blended. Fold in the chicken. Let marinate while you prepare the sauce.

Lightly coat a medium nonstick skillet with cooking spray and place over medium-low heat. Add the onion and cauliflower and cook for 5 minutes, stirring, until softened. Add the ginger and tomato sauce and reduce the heat to low.

Meanwhile, place the chicken on an aluminum-foil-lined baking sheet and broil just until lightly charred in spots, about 5 minutes. Flip the chicken and broil for 3 more minutes, or until cooked through. Using tongs, lift the chicken off the baking sheet and add to the sauce, still over medium-low heat. Stir to coat the chicken and warm through. Remove from the heat, stir in the remaining about 1/2 cup yogurt, season with salt and pepper to taste, and serve with the warm rice.

<u>Nutritional analysis:</u> Calories 434, carbohydrates 60 grams, protein 32 grams, fat 5 grams Carbs 58%, protein 31%, fat 11%

SNACKS

ALMONDS

Almonds are especially satisfying and impart a whole host of health benefits. Just a palmful of almonds contains loads of protein and healthy fats. Scientific studies have shown that eating almonds can lead to mild reductions in LDL cholesterol (the bad kind) and can potentially reduce the risk of heart disease. Aim for about 20 to 25 almonds for your snack.

APPLE AND NUT BUTTER

Peanut, almond, sunflower—your snack, your choice! Just remember portion control. Add a dollop of nut butter to a bowl with your sliced apple, close the nut butter jar, and leave the kitchen.

CHEESE AND CRACKERS

There are so many varieties of crackers in the stores—it can be a bit overwhelming. My suggestion is to take a few minutes to read the nutritional information on the package. Look for high-fiber, no-sugar options. My favorites are Finn Crisp, Wasa, and Mary's Gone Crackers (which are gluten-free). Slice up about 1 ounce (or about 2 thin slices) of reduced-fat cheese (or one slice of full-fat cheese) for a topping.

POPCORN

Popcorn is such a fun snack. Again, review the nutrition facts before purchasing. Look for high-fiber, low- (or no-) sugar varieties and fewer than 150 calories per serving. Better yet, pop your own using whole kernels, either on the stovetop, in a microwave bowl, or in an air popper. Aim for about 5 cups for a snack serving.

JICAMA AND LIME

Go ahead—try a new vegetable! Jicama is a crunchy root veggie that tastes a bit like an apple but not as sweet. To serve, peel off the tough brown skin and cut it into slices or matchsticks. For a cool, crisp snack, I like to drizzle slices with fresh lime juice. Half a jicama will yield about 3 cups of slices. It's also a great addition to a salad.

TURKEY AND PICKLE PLATTER

High-protein, low-fat sliced turkey and sliced pickles make for a savory and energy-boosting snack. Serving suggestion: 2 to 3 ounces sliced turkey and all the pickles you want.

EDAMAME

A nutritional powerhouse, loaded with protein, fiber, and healthy fats, this soybean is available both fresh (look for vacuum-packed bags at Trader Joe's) and frozen. I like to keep a bag in the freezer to pull out and toss into stir-fries and soups. For snacking, either boil or microwave to warm up a handful.

HOMEMADE HUMMUS

MAKES 2 CUPS

Of course, you can buy premade hummus at the store, but it's so quick and easy to make it at home. Plus, you know exactly what is in the dish. Tahini, a paste made from ground sesame seeds, is a great source of healthy fats.

HARLEY HACK: It's annoying to use only part of a can of beans; that's why you're making a full batch of hummus. It will keep in the fridge for at least a week.

1 can (15 ounces) chickpeas, drained

1/2 cup tahini

2 tablespoons fresh lemon juice or bottled lemon concentrate, plus more to taste

1/2 teaspoon salt, plus more to taste

Sliced vegetables of your choice (such as carrots, cucumbers, bell peppers, or tomatoes)

Place the chickpeas in the bowl of a food processor and blend for 1 minute, or until the mixture forms clumps. Scrape down the sides of the bowl, then add the tahini, lemon juice, and salt and blend until pureed. With the machine running, pour in up to 1/4 cup water, 1 tablespoon at a time, until the mixture is creamy. Taste and add salt and/or water, if needed.

To serve, scoop 1/4 cup hummus onto a plate. Arrange the vegetables around the hummus and drizzle with additional lemon juice, if desired.

Nutritional analysis (for 1/4 cup hummus): Calories 126, carbohydrates 16 grams, protein 6 grams, fat 4 grams
Carbs 50%, protein 20%, fat 30%

DECONSTRUCTED BERRY COBBLER

SERVES 1

Fresh or frozen strawberries, blackberries, raspberries, blueberries? All work. Hazelnuts, almonds, or pecans? Your choice. Just make sure to opt for nonfat yogurt—you'll get lots of healthy fat from the nuts.

1 cup nonfat plain Greek yogurt

1/2 cup low-sugar muesli cereal (not granola)

3/4 cup fresh or thawed frozen mixed berries of your choice

2 tablespoons chopped hazelnuts or nut of your choice

Spoon the yogurt, muesli, and berries in alternating layers in a parfait or tall wide glass. Top with the nuts and serve immediately.

Nutritional analysis: Calories 395, carbohydrates 53 grams, protein 29 grams, fat 11 grams Carbs 50%, protein 27%, fat 23%

CRACKERS WITH SMOKED SALMON AND HERBED YOGURT

SERVES 1

Make a snack feel special by topping hearty crackers and salmon slices with a creamy, herby dip.

HARLEY HACK: Snacks are meant to be quick, but take the time to place this little meal on a plate and sit down to eat it. You will enjoy it more and there is less opportunity to mindlessly overeat.

¼ cup nonfat plain Greek yogurt

2 tablespoons chopped fresh flat-leaf parsley, tarragon, dill, or chives

1 ounce smoked salmon, cut into small slices

3 whole-grain high-fiber crackers

Combine the yogurt and chopped herbs in a small bowl. Arrange the salmon over the crackers and top with the herbed yogurt to serve.

Nutritional analysis: Calories 135, carbohydrates 24 grams, protein 8 grams, fat 5 grams
Carbs 69%, protein 24%, fat 7%

HARLEY GUACAMOLE

MAKES 1¾ CUPS; 2 SERVINGS

Avocado is a great source of healthy fat, and it makes for a quick dip or a wonderful spread on toast or sandwiches. This recipe includes protein-rich edamame and makes enough for two servings, so share with friends or bring leftovers into work for appreciative co-workers!

HARLEY HACK: Remember the seeds of the jalapeño bring the heat, so leave them out if you don't like things spicy. If cilantro isn't to your taste, leave it out.

¾ cup fresh or thawed frozen shelled edamame

1 small ripe avocado, peeled and pitted (about ½ cup flesh)

1 garlic clove, minced (optional)

2 tablespoons fresh lime juice or bottled lime concentrate

1 tablespoon minced jalapeño pepper (optional)

¼ cup chopped fresh cilantro (optional)

Salt and freshly ground black pepper

1 high-fiber tortilla

Carrot slices, cherry tomatoes, or radish slices for garnish (optional)

Combine the edamame, avocado, garlic (if using), and lime juice in a food processor or blender and process until smooth, thinning with water to the desired consistency. Spoon the mixture into a serving bowl, fold in the jalapeño and cilantro (if using), and season with salt and pepper to taste.

Toast the tortilla in a toaster oven or in a hot skillet until lightly browned and crisp. Break into pieces and serve with the guacamole and veggies (if using).

Nutritional analysis: Calories 150, carbohydrates 16 grams, protein 10 grams, fat 9 grams
Carbs 35%, protein 21%, fat 43%

The Path Ahead

Good health is for *everybody*. Feeling healthy, looking lean, having energy, and being strong enough to live your life on your own terms should be available to all. There is no perfect diet or perfect supplement, but there are effective ways of eating that can give you the nutrition you need, no matter your budget, food preferences, schedule, or lifestyle.

The Carb Reset is a step toward sustainable behaviors that help you *store less fat* and *burn more fat*. Focusing on only one side of the equation will push you toward the extremes that have likely been the cause of your past frustrations. *The Carb Reset* is about giving yourself a chance to start over, shake off the deprivation of other diets, and allow your past failures to become distant memories, so your current and future successes will allow you to see yourself more positively.

I hope this book has lifted the curtain and shown you that every diet for the last forty years is essentially the same thing repackaged with focus on a different problem. You don't need to bounce from diet to diet. You simply need to identify what foods you enjoy, make a time and place for them, and then use PATH to fill your meals with nutritious foods that will fuel your everyday life.

The foods that form the foundation of PATH don't need to be exotic and expensive. They are the frozen berries you can buy in the grocery store, the beans that come in a can, the lean poultry or fish you can order affordably online, and the pasta or rice you can buy for a couple of dollars.

Weight loss has always felt hard because we've made it hard. It's a bumpy road filled with roadblocks, hurdles, and ditches. Unfortunately, those obstacles have been created by the diet industry that was supposed to give you an exit from your dietary struggles but led you only further astray.

I've spent thirty years helping people become healthier by avoiding the misleading information that sends them on a detour that keeps them working hard without seeing results. And I'll spend the rest of my days trying to give people peace of mind that they, too, can have the body and life they want.

Your body is fine the way it is. What's broken is the way you've been taught to eat. If I can promise you anything, it's that you won't regret this new path toward health. It's everything those other diets promise— balanced, sustainable, and effective—but without the lies, deception, and difficulty.

When you're on the right path, everything feels different. It feels *right*. No one has ever regretted a great meal. You don't see people being upset about eating sushi, pasta, and dessert. You see people avoiding those things because they're told they can't have them.

No one enjoys taking fat-loss pills, drinking weight-loss teas, and following the latest starvation detox plan. People do them because they think there is no other way to lose weight and gain health. I hope you now know there is another way, and it can be more enjoyable and balanced than you were ever told.

I've made a lot of mistakes in my time. Even I fell for SnackWell's. But one day you either realize that change happens with consistent healthy behaviors, or you keep doing things you know don't feel good, even though they never deliver the changes you desire.

This book has been decades in the making. It brings together the analysis of dozens of game-changing studies with my longtime real-life experience. It's the healthiest nutrition advice and lifestyle habits all wrapped up into one easy-to-follow plan. It's a plan that helps you think less and act more.

The best part? Unlike with other diet plans, you don't have to suffer to succeed. You just need to be willing to reset your mind, body, and commitment to avoiding tempting (but misleading) trends and headlines. And if you lose your way, don't get discouraged. This diet is flexible, and it's easy to reset and start your journey again.

By shifting your perspective—and adding carbs back into your life—you will eat better and feel better. That's when you know you've reached the road to long-lasting health. Once you're on the PATH, keep your eyes ahead and don't ever look back.

Endnotes

CHAPTER 1: THE TRUTH ABOUT LOSING WEIGHT

1. As I write this today, the obesity rate: Centers for Disease Control, "Adult Obesity Facts," May 14, 2024, https://www.cdc.gov/obesity/php/data -research/adult-obesity-facts.html.

2. Global weight gain: World Obesity Atlas, "Economic impact of over-weight and obesity to surpass $4 trillion by 2035," 2023, https://www .worldobesity.org/news/economic-impact-of-overweight-and-obesity -to-surpass-4-trillion-by-2035.

3. Haub lost twenty-seven pounds: NPR staff, "Professor's Weight Loss Secret: Junk Food," NPR, November 13, 2010, https://www.npr.org/ 2010/11/12/131286626/professor-s-weight-loss-secret-junk-food.

4. After all, less than 20 percent: Rena R. Wing and Suzanne Phelan, "Long-term weight loss maintenance," *American Journal of Clinical Nutrition* 82 (Suppl.) (2005): 222S–25S. https://ajcn.nutrition.org/article/ S0002-9165(23)29536-2/fulltext.

5. As long as caloric balance: Brad Jon Schoenfeld, Alan Albert Aragon, and James W. Krieger, "Effects of meal frequency on weight loss and body composition: a meta-analysis," *Nutrition Reviews* 73, no. 2 (February 2015): 69–82. https://academic.oup.com/nutritionreviews/article/73/2/ 69/1820875.

6. Findings indicated no significant differences: Ruth Schübel, Johanna Nattenmüller, Disorn Sookthai, Tobias Nonnenmacher, Mirja E. Graf, Lena Riedl et al., "Effects of intermittent and continuous calorie restriction on body weight and metabolism over 50 wk: a randomized controlled trial," *American Journal of Clinical Nutrition* (November 2018). https://ajcn .nutrition.org/article/S0002-9165(22)03026-X/fulltext.

7. Long-term studies: Longitudinal studies: Tatiana Moro, Grant Tinsley, Antonino Bianco, Giuseppe Marcolin, Quirico Francesco Pacelli, Giuseppe Battaglia et al., "Effects of eight weeks of time-restricted feeding (16/8) on basal metabolism, maximal strength, body composition, inflammation, and cardiovascular risk factors in resistance-trained males," *Journal of Translational Medicine* 14, no. 1 (Oct. 13, 2016): 290. doi: 10.1186/s12967-016-1044-0. PMID: 27737674; PMCID: PMC5064803. https://pubmed.ncbi.nlm.nih.gov/27737674/.

8. Impact on physical performance: Studies: Grant M. Tinsley, Jeffrey S. Forsse, Natalie K. Butler, Antonio Paoli, Annie A. Bane, Paul M. La Bounty et al., "Time-restricted feeding in young men performing resistance training: a randomized controlled trial," *European Journal of Sport Science* 17, no. 2 (Mar. 2017): 200–207. doi: 10.1080/17461391.2016.1223173. PMID: 27550719. https://pubmed.ncbi.nlm.nih.gov/27550719/.

9. Individual variability: Recent research: K. A. Varady, D. J. Roohk, Y. C. Loe, B. K. McEvoy-Hein, and M. K. Hellerstein, "Effects of modified alternate-day fasting regimens on adipocyte size, triglyceride metabolism, and plasma adiponectin levels in mice," *Journal of Lipid Research* 48, no. 10 (Oct. 2007): 2212–19. doi: 10.1194/jlr.M700223-JLR200. Epub 2007 Jul 2. PMID: 17607017. https://pubmed.ncbi.nlm.nih.gov/17607017/.

CHAPTER 2: PATH: AN EATING PLAN THAT FITS IN THE PALM OF YOUR HAND

1. In a yearlong, randomized clinical: Christopher D. Gardner, John F. Trepanowski, Liana C. Del Gobbo et al., "Effect of low-fat vs. low-carbohydrate diet on 12-month weight loss in overweight adults and the association with genotype pattern or insulin secretion: the DIETFITS randomized clinical trial," *JAMA* 319, no. 7 (2018): 667–69. doi: 10.1001/jama.2018.0245. https://jamanetwork.com/journals/jama/fullarticle/2673150.

CHAPTER 3: SKINNY PEOPLE EAT BREAD (AND OTHER DELICIOUS CARBS)

1. For this reason, it is sometimes: A. B. Jenkins, T. P. Markovic, A. Fleury, and L. V. Campbell, "Carbohydrate intake and short-term regulation of leptin in humans," *Diabetologia* 40, no. 3 (1997): 348–51. doi: 10.1007/s001250050686. PMID: 9084976. https://pubmed.ncbi.nlm.nih.gov/9084976/.

2. Research suggests that your cortisol: L. Tsai, J. Karpakka, C. Aginger, C. Johansson, A. Pousette, and K. Carlström, "Basal concentrations of anabolic and catabolic hormones in relation to endurance exercise after short-term changes in diet," *European Journal of Applied Physiology and Occupational Physiology* 66, no. 4 (1993): 304–8. doi: 10.1007/BF00237773. PMID: 8495690. https://pubmed.ncbi.nlm.nih.gov/8495690/.

3. Over the last ten years, there has: Seung Hee Lee, Latetia V. Moore, So-hyun Park, Diane M. Harris, and Heidi M. Blanck, "Adults Meeting Fruit and Vegetable Intake Recommendations—United States, 2019," *Morbidity and Mortality Weekly Report (MMWR)* 71 (2022). https://www.cdc.gov/mmwr/volumes/71/wr/pdfs/mm7101a1-H.pdf.

4. But a 2021 review of more: Ellen E. Blaak, Gabriele Riccardi, and Leslie Cho, "Carbohydrates: separating fact from fiction," *Atherosclerosis*, March 27, 2021. doi: https://doi.org/10.1016/j.atherosclerosis.2021.03.025. https://www.atherosclerosis-journal.com/article/S0021-9150(21)00146-5/abstract.

5. According to research published in *Clinical Nutrition*: Viviana Loria-Kohen, Carmen Gómez-Candela, Ceila Fernández-Fernández, Almudena Pérez-Torres, Juan García-Puig, and Laura M. Bermejo, "Evaluation of the usefulness of a low-calorie diet with or without bread in the treatment of overweight/obesity," *Clinical Nutrition*, December 19, 2011. doi: https://doi.org/10.1016/j.clnu.2011.12.002. https://www.clinicalnutritionjournal.com/article/S0261-5614(11)00233-0/abstract#secd36576611e964.

6. In an analysis of the diets of more: Mengna Huang, Kenneth Lo, Jie Li, Matthew Allison, Wen-Chih Wu, Simin Liu et al., "Pasta meal intake in relation to risks of type 2 diabetes and atherosclerotic cardiovascular disease in postmenopausal women: findings from the Women's Health Initiative," *BMJ Nutrition, Prevention & Health* 4 (2021). doi: 10.1136/bmjnph-2020-000198. https://nutrition.bmj.com/content/4/1/195.

7. One study suggests that: Dagfinn Aune, NaNa Keum, Edward Giovannucci, Lars T. Fadnes, Paolo Boffetta, Darren C. Greenwood, Serena Tonstad, Lars J. Vatten, Elio Riboli, Teresa Norat, "Whole grain consumption and risk of cardiovascular disease, cancer, and all cause and cause specific mortality: systematic review and dose-response meta-analysis of prospective studies," *BMJ*, June 14, 2016, https://pmc.ncbi.nlm.nih.gov/articles/PMC4908315/.

8. Bread is an integral piece of the Mediterranean: Antonia Trichopoulou, Miguel A. Martínez-González, Tammy Y. N. Tong, Nita G. Forhoui, Shweta Khandelwal, Dorairaj Prabhakaran et al., "Definitions and potential health benefits of the Mediterranean diet: views from experts around the world," *BMC Medicine* 12, no. 112 (2014). https://doi.org/10.1186/1741-7015-12-112; https://bmcmedicine.biomedcentral.com/articles/10.1186/1741-7015-12-112.

9. If you need help finding the best: Rebecca S. Mozaffarian, Rebekka M. Lee, Mary A. Kennedy, David S. Ludwig, Dariush Mozaffarian, and Steven L. Gortmaker, "Identifying whole grain foods: a comparison of

different approaches for selecting more healthful whole grain products," *Public Health Nutrition* 16, no. 12 (Dec. 2013): 2255–64. doi: 10.1017/S1 368980012005447. PMID: 23286205; PMCID: PMC4486284. https:// www.ncbi.nlm.nih.gov/pmc/articles/PMC4486284/.

10. Here are some tasty and healthy: Kerry Torrens, "Top 10 healthiest breads," goodFOOD, March 15, 2023, https://www.bbcgoodfood.com/ howto/guide/what-is-the-healthiest-bread.

11. The Mediterranean diet, which has: Harvard T. H. Chan School of Public Health, The Nutrition Source, "Diet Review: Mediterranean Diet," April 2023, https://nutritionsource.hsph.harvard.edu/healthy-weight/ diet-reviews/mediterranean-diet/.

CHAPTER 4: ALL VEGGIES, ALL THE TIME

1. A study found that "phytochemicals . . .": Dhandevi Pem and Rajesh Jeewon, "Fruit and vegetable intake: benefits and progress of nutrition education interventions—narrative review article," *Iranian Journal of Public Health* 44, no. 10 (Oct. 2015): 1309–21. PMID: 26576343; PMCID: PMC4644575. https://www.ncbi.nlm.nih.gov/pmc/articles/ PMC4644575/.

2. A study from the Mayo Clinic found: Lisa Hayes, M.D., "What's the deal with probiotics?" Mayo Clinic Health System, September 15, 2021, https://www.mayoclinichealthsystem.org/hometown-health/speaking -of-health/whats-the-deal-with-probiotics.

3. Eating more fruits and vegetables: Heidi Godman, "How many fruits and vegetables do we really need?" Harvard Health Publishing, September 1, 2021, https://www.health.harvard.edu/nutrition/how-many-fruits-and -vegetables-do-we-really-need.

4. According to the American Diabetes Association: Rani Polak, Edward M. Phillips, and Amy Campbell, "Legumes: health benefits and culinary approaches to increase intake," *Clinical Diabetes* 33, no. 4 (Oct. 2015): 198–205. doi: 10.2337/diaclin.33.4.198. PMID: 26487796; PMCID: PMC4608274. https://www.ncbi.nlm.nih.gov/pmc/articles/ PMC4608274/.

5. Eating beans can be good: Ibid.

6. A study in *Advances in Nutrition* found: Nikan Zargarzadeh, Seyed Mohammad Mousavi, Heitor O. Santos, Daggfin Aune, Shirin Hasani-Ranjbar, Bagher Larijani et al., "Legume consumption and risk of all-cause and cause-specific mortality: a systematic review and dose-response meta-analysis of prospective studies," *Advances in Nutrition* 14, no. 1 (Jan. 2023): 64–76. doi: 10.1016/j.advnut.2022.10.009. Epub 2023 Jan 5. PMID:

36811595; PMCID: PMC10103007. https://pubmed.ncbi.nlm.nih.gov/36811595/.

CHAPTER 5: FAT FACTS

1. That's *a lot* of added calories: Hodan Farah Wells and Jean C. Buzby, "Dietary Assessment of Major Trends in U.S. Food Consumption, 1970–2005," *Economic Information Bulletin*, no. 33 (March 2008). Economic Research Service, U.S. Dept. of Agriculture. https://www.ers.usda.gov/webdocs/publications/44217/eib-33.pdf?v=1.9.

2. To give you an idea of what many: Linda Kantor and Andrzej Blazejczyk, "Food Availability (Per Capita) Data System," USDA Economic Research Service, September 27, 2024, https://www.ers.usda.gov/data-products/food-availability-per-capita-data-system/food-availability-per-capita-data-system/#Loss-Adjusted%20Food%20Availability.

3. A twenty-five-year study: Henry N. Ginsberg and Paul R. MacCallum, "The obesity, metabolic syndrome, and type 2 diabetes mellitus pandemic: part I. Increased cardiovascular disease risk and the importance of atherogenic dyslipidemia in persons with the metabolic syndrome and type 2 diabetes mellitus," *Journal of the CardioMetabolic Syndrome* 4, no. 2 (Spring 2009): 113–19. doi: 10.1111/j.1559-4572.2008.00044.x. PMID: 19614799; PMCID: PMC2901596. https://www.ncbi.nlm.nih.gov/pmc/articles/PMC2901596/.

4. In fact, in one study of more than: American College of Cardiology, "Unsaturated fats, high-quality carbs lower risk of heart disease," *ScienceDaily*, September 28, 2015. https://www.sciencedaily.com/releases/2015/09/150928144025.htm (accessed August 19, 2024).

5. A study called the: Ramón Estruch, Emilio Ros, Jordi Salas-Salvadó, Maria-Isabel Covas, Dolores Corella, Fernando Arós et al., "Primary prevention of cardiovascular disease with a Mediterranean diet supplemented with extra-virgin olive oil or nuts," *New England Journal of Medicine* 378 (June 21, 2018): e34. doi: 10.1056/NEJMoa1800389. https://www.nejm.org/doi/full/10.1056/NEJMoa1800389.

6. A perfect example is coconut oil: Michael Shilling, Laurie Matt, Evelyn Rubin, Mark Paul Visitacion, Nairmeen A. Haller, Scott F. Grey et al., "Antimicrobial effects of virgin coconut oil and its medium-chain fatty acids on *Clostridium difficile*," *Journal of Medicinal Food* 16, no. 12 (Dec. 2013): 1079–85. doi: 10.1089/jmf.2012.0303. PMID: 24328700. https://pubmed.ncbi.nlm.nih.gov/24328700/.

7. One study showed that men: Marie-Pierre St.-Onge, Robert Ross, William D. Parsons, and Peter J. H. Jones, "Medium-chain triglycerides

increase energy expenditure and decrease adiposity in overweight men," *Obesity Research* 11 (2003): 395–402. https://doi.org/10.1038/oby.2003 .53; https://onlinelibrary.wiley.com/doi/full/10.1038/oby.2003.53.

8. If that wasn't enough to make you: Flávia Xavier Valente, Flávia Galvão Cândido, Lílian Lelis Lopes, Desirrê Morais Dias, Samantha Dalbosco, Lins Carvalho et al., "Effects of coconut oil consumption on energy metabolism, cardiometabolic risk markers, and appetitive responses in women with excess body fat," *European Journal of Nutrition* 57 (2018): 1627–37. https://doi.org/10.1007/s00394-017-1448-5; https://link.springer.com/ article/10.1007/s00394-017-1448-5.

9. Coconut oil's glowing reputation: Frank M. Sacks, Alice H. Lichtenstein, Jason H. Y. Wu, Lawrence J. Appel, Mark A. Creager, Penny M. Kris-Etherton et al., "Dietary Fats and Cardiovascular Disease: A Presidential Advisory from the American Heart Association," https://www .ahajournals.org/doi/10.1161/CIR.0000000000000510#sec-10.

10. And while saturated fat has: Jillian Kubala, MS, RD, "Is Saturated Fat Unhealthy?" Healthline, December 19, 2023, https://www.healthline .com/nutrition/saturated-fat.

11. Additionally, a review of fourteen different: A. C. Rego Costa, E. L. Rosado, and M. Soares-Mota, "Influence of the dietary intake of medium chain triglycerides on body composition, energy expenditure and satiety: a systematic review," *Nutrición Hospitalaria* 27, no. 1 (Jan.–Feb. 2012): 103–8. doi: 10.1590/S0212-16112012000100011. PMID: 22566308. https://pubmed.ncbi.nlm.nih.gov/22566308/.

12. Research in forty-two studies found: Mojgan Amiri, Hamidreza Raeisi-Dehkordi, Nizal Sarrafzadegan, Scott C. Forbes, and Amin Salehi-Abargouei, "The effects of canola oil on cardiovascular risk factors: a systematic review and meta-analysis with dose-response analysis of controlled clinical trials," *Nutrition, Metabolism and Cardiovascular Diseases* 30, no. 12 (Nov. 27, 2020): 2133–45. doi: 10.1016/j.numecd.2020.06.007. Epub 2020 Jun 18. PMID: 33127255. https://pubmed.ncbi.nlm.nih.gov/ 33127255/.

13. Much of the concern regarding the omega-6: Jacqueline K. Innes and Philip C. Calder, "Omega-6 fatty acids and inflammation," *PLEFA*, March 22, 2018. doi: https://doi.org/10.1016/j.plefa.2018.03.004; https://www.plefa.com/article/S0952-3278(18)30074-7/abstract?mc _cid=339a479773&mc_cid=80b964a3d2&mc_eid=44e8861a4a&mc_eid =44e8861a4a.

14. A word (or two) on saturated fat: Nina Teicholz, "A short history of saturated fat: the making and unmaking of a scientific consensus," *Current Opinion in Endocrinology, Diabetes and Obesity* 30, no. 1 (Feb. 1,

2023): 65–71. doi: 10.1097/MED.0000000000000791. PMID: 36477384; PMCID: PMC9794145. https://www.ncbi.nlm.nih.gov/pmc/articles/PMC9794145/.

CHAPTER 6: PROTEIN POWER

1. An article in the *Journal of Obesity*: Jaecheol Moon and Gwanpyo Koh, "Clinical evidence and mechanisms of high-protein diet-induced weight loss," *Journal of Obesity & Metabolic Syndrome* 29, no. 3 (Sept. 30, 2020): 166–73. doi: 10.7570/jomes20028. PMID: 32699189; PMCID: PMC7539343. https://pubmed.ncbi.nlm.nih.gov/32699189/.

2. Consuming protein can also have: Heather J. Leidy, Minghua Tang, Cheryl L. H. Armstrong, Carmen B. Martin, and Wayne W. Campbell, "The effects of consuming frequent, higher protein meals on appetite and satiety during weight loss in overweight/obese men," *Obesity* (Silver Spring, Md.) 19, no. 4 (Apr. 2011): 818–24. doi: 10.1038/oby.2010.203. Epub 2010 Sep 16. PMID: 20847729; PMCID: PMC4564867. https://pubmed.ncbi.nlm.nih.gov/20847729/.

3. It does not take as much energy: Deanna Pai, "Can Eating More Protein Help You Lose Weight? Here's What the Science Says," EatingWell, June 16, 2024, https://www.eatingwell.com/article/7913417/can-eating-more-protein-help-you-lose-weight/.

4. There is also a strong link between: Barath Prashanth Sivasubramanian, Mihir Dave, Viraj Panchal, Johnnie Saifa-Bonsu, Srujana Konka, Farahnaz Noei et al., "Comprehensive review of red meat consumption and the risk of cancer," *Cureus: Journal of Medical Science* 15, no. 9 (Sept. 15, 2023): e45324. doi: 10.7759/cureus.45324. PMID: 37849565; PMCID: PMC10577092. https://www.ncbi.nlm.nih.gov/pmc/articles/PMC10577092/.

5. Too much sodium has been: Lizzie Streit, MS, RDN, LD, Kris Gunnars, BSc, and Rachael Ajmera, MS, R, "Does Red Meat Have Health Benefits? A Look at the Science," Healthline, April 26, 2023, https://www.healthline.com/nutrition/is-red-meat-bad-for-you-or-good#nutrition.

6. Other seafood such as salmon: John Donovan, "The Health Benefits of Salmon," WebMD, August 8, 2023, https://www.webmd.com/food-recipes/benefits-salmon.

7. If you miss the taste of meat: Emily Gelsomin, MLA, RD, LDN, "Impossible and Beyond: How healthy are these meatless burgers?" Harvard Health Publishing/Harvard Medical School, January 24, 2022, https://www.health.harvard.edu/blog/impossible-and-beyond-how-healthy-are-these-meatless-burgers-2019081517448.

8. Great Sources of Protein: Jenette Restivo, "High-protein foods: The best

protein sources to include in a healthy diet," Harvard Health Publishing/ Harvard Medical School, December 1, 2023, https://www.health.harvard .edu/nutrition/high-protein-foods-the-best-protein-sources-to-include -in-a-healthy-diet.

9. Great Sources of Protein: Natalie Rizzo, MS, RD, "6 High-Protein Grains to Add to Your Pantry, According to a Dietitian," EatingWell, https://www.eatingwell.com/article/8049010/high-protein-grains-to -add-to-your-pantry/.

10. Great Sources of Protein: American Heart Association/Health for Good, "Plant-based Protein Sources," April 22, 2024, https://www.heart.org/ en/healthy-living/healthy-eating/eat-smart/nutrition-basics/plant-based -protein-infographic.

CHAPTER 7: THE SCOOP ON SUGAR

1. Sugar becomes a problem when: C. Rob Markus, Peter J. Rogers, Fred Brouns, and Robbie Schepers, "Eating dependence and weight gain; no human evidence for a 'sugar-addiction' model of overweight," *Appetite,* July 1, 2017. https://www.sciencedirect.com/science/article/abs/pii/ S0195666317304099.

2. You can drink and drink and: An Pan and Frank B. Hu, "Effects of carbohydrates on satiety: differences between liquid and solid food," *Current Opinion in Clinical Nutrition & Metabolic Care* 14, no. 4 (July 2011): 385– 90. doi: 10.1097/MCO.0b013e328346df36. PMID: 21519237. https:// pubmed.ncbi.nlm.nih.gov/21519237/.

3. Perhaps it's unsurprising that soft: Vasanti S. Malik, Matthias B. Schulze, and Frank B. Hu, "Intake of sugar-sweetened beverages and weight gain: a systematic review," *American Journal of Clinical Nutrition* 84, no. 2 (Aug. 2006): 274–88. doi: 10.1093/ajcn/84.1.274. PMID: 16895873; PMCID: PMC3210834. https://www.ncbi.nlm.nih.gov/pmc/articles/ PMC3210834/.

4. In a recent study, participants: Fabrice Bonnet, Aude Tavenard, Maxime Esvan, Bruno Laviolle, Mélanie Viltard, Eve M. Lepicard et al., "Consumption of a carbonated beverage with high-intensity sweeteners has no effect on insulin sensitivity and secretion in nondiabetic adults," *Journal of Nutrition* 148, no. 8 (August 2018): 1293–99. https://jn.nutrition.org/ article/S0022-3166(22)16379-0/fulltext#secsect0005.

5. They conducted a meta-analysis: Ingrid Toews, Szimonetta Lohner, Daniela Küllenberg de Gaudry, Harriet Sommer, and Joerg J. Meerpohl, "Association between intake of non-sugar sweeteners and health outcomes: systematic review and meta-analyses of randomised and non-randomised

controlled trials and observational studies," *BMJ* 364 (2019): k4718. doi: 10.1136/bmj.k4718. https://www.bmj.com/content/364/bmj.k4718.

6. Some recent studies have also: Kamal Patel, "Did You Know That Sugary Fruits Could Help Regulate . . . Blood Sugar?" Examine, January 31, 2023, https://examine.com/articles/did-you-know-sugary-fruit-could -help-regulate-blood-sugar/.

7. If you ate an orange instead: Stanford Medicine Children's Health, "Fruit vs. Fruit Juice: What's the Difference?" https://www.stanfordchildrens .org/en/topic/default?id=fruit-vs-fruit-juice-whats-the-difference-197 -30060.

8. One study investigated what happens: D. J. Jenkins, C. W. Kendall, D. G. Popovich, E. Vidgen, C. C. Mehling, V. Vuksan et al., "Effect of a very-high-fiber vegetable, fruit, and nut diet on serum lipids and colonic function," *Metabolism* 50, no. 4 (Apr. 2001): 494–503. doi: 10.1053/ meta.2001.21037. PMID: 11288049. https://pubmed.ncbi.nlm.nih.gov/ 11288049/.

9. All fruits are good for you: Mayo Clinic Staff, "Chart of high-fiber foods," Mayo Clinic, Healthy Lifestyle, Nutrition and Healthy Eating, November 23, 2023, https://www.mayoclinic.org/healthy-lifestyle/ nutrition-and-healthy-eating/in-depth/high-fiber-foods/art-20050948.

CHAPTER 8: PERSONALIZING YOUR PATH

1. Reduced risk of obesity: People: Amber A.W.A. van der Heijden, Frank B. Hu, Eric Rimm, and Rob van Dam, "A prospective study of breakfast consumption and weight gain among U.S. men," *Obesity* (Silver Spring, Md.) 15, no. 10 (2007). 2463–69. doi: 10.1038/oby.2007.292. https:// www.researchgate.net/publication/5920517_A_Prospective_Study_of _Breakfast_Consumption_and_Weight_Gain_among_US_Men.

2. Improved metabolism: Eating: James A. Betts, Enhad A. Chowdhury, Javier T. Gonzalez, Judith D. Richardson, Kostas Tsintzas, and Dylan Thompson, "Is breakfast the most important meal of the day?" *Proceedings of the Nutrition Society* 75, no. 4 (2016): 464–74. doi: 10.1017/ S0029665116000318. https://www.cambridge.org/core/journals/ proceedings-of-the-nutrition-society/article/is-breakfast-the-most -important-meal-of-the-day/74DC8BF20CAF1D7D5E75CD46 A35451F8.

3. Better nutrient intake: Breakfast eaters: Priya Deshmukh-Taskar, John Radcliffe, Yan Liu, and Theresa Nicklas, "Do breakfast skipping and breakfast type affect energy intake, nutrient intake, nutrient adequacy, and diet quality in young adults? NHANES 1999–2002," *Journal of the*

American College of Nutrition 29, no. 4 (2010): 407–18. doi: https://doi .org/10.1080/07315724.2010.10719858.

4. Enhanced cognitive function: Breakfast: Gail C. Rampersaud, Mark A. Pereira, Beverly L. Girard, Judi Adams, and Jordan D. Metzl, "Breakfast habits, nutritional status, body weight, and academic performance in children and adolescents," *Journal of the American Dietetic Association* 105, no. 5 (May 2005): 743–60; quiz 761–62. doi: 10.1016/j.jada.2005.02.007. PMID: 15883552. https://pubmed.ncbi.nlm.nih.gov/15883552/.

5. Stable blood sugar levels: Eating: Andrew O. Odegaard, David R. Jacobs, Jr., Lyn M. Steffen, Linda Van Horn, David S. Ludwig, and Mark A. Pereira, "Breakfast frequency and development of metabolic risk," *Diabetes Care* 36, no. 10 (Oct. 2013): 3100–106. doi: 10.2337/dc13-0316. PMID: 23775814; PMCID: PMC3781522. https://diabetesjournals.org/ care/article/36/10/3100/30090/Breakfast-Frequency-and-Development -of-Metabolic.

6. Improved appetite control: Careful: Heather J. Leidy, Cheryl L. H. Armstrong, Minghua Tang, Richard D. Mattes, and Wayne W. Campbell, "The influence of higher protein intake and greater eating frequency on appetite control in overweight and obese men," *Obesity* (Silver Spring, Md.) 18, no. 9 (Sept. 2010): 1725–32. doi: 10.1038/oby.2010.45. PMID: 20339363; PMCID: PMC4034047. https://pubmed.ncbi.nlm.nih.gov/ 20339363/.

7. Maintaining metabolic rate: Eating: F. Bellisle, R. McDevitt, and A. M. Prentice, "Meal frequency and energy balance," *British Journal of Nutrition* 77, Suppl. 1 (Apr. 1997): S57–S70. doi: 10.1079/bjn19970104. PMID: 9155494. https://pubmed.ncbi.nlm.nih.gov/9155494/.

8. Balanced blood sugar levels: Healthy: David J. A. Jenkins, Thomas M. S. Wolever, Vladimir Vuksan, Furio Brighenti, Stephen C. Cunnane, A. Venketeshwer Rao et al., "Nibbling versus gorging: metabolic advantages of increased meal frequency," *New England Journal of Medicine* 321 (Oct. 5, 1989): 929–34. doi: 10.1056/NEJM198910053211403.

9. Enhanced nutrient intake: Nutrient-dense: M. Vadiveloo, H. Parker, and H. Raynor, "Increasing low-energy-dense foods and decreasing high-energy-dense foods differently influence weight loss trial outcomes," *International Journal of Obesity* 42 (2018): 479–86.

10. Behavioral control: Planning and consuming: Jean Kristeller, Yann Cornil, France Bellisle, and Sophie Vinoy, "Mindful Eating Applied to Snacking: A Promising Behavioral Approach Supported by Research. Summary of the Symposium Held at the 21st International Congress of Nutrition (IUNS 2017)," *Journal of Human Nutrition and Food Science* 8, no. 1 (2020):

1131. https://www.jscimedcentral.com/public/assets/articles/nutrition
-8-1131.pdf.

11. Research shows that snackers who: Santiago Navas-Carretero, Itziar
Abete, M. Angeles Zulet, and J. Alfredo Martínez, "Chronologically
scheduled snacking with high-protein products within the habitual diet
in type-2 diabetes patients leads to a fat mass loss: a longitudinal study,"
Nutrition Journal 10 (July 14, 2011): 74. doi: 10.1186/1475-2891-10-74.
PMID: 21756320; PMCID: PMC3155966. https://pubmed.ncbi.nlm
.nih.gov/21756320/.

12. Research shows that portion sizes: NIH, We Can! ® Community News
Feature, "Larger Portion Sizes Contribute to U.S. Obesity Problem," February 13, 2013, https://www.nhlbi.nih.gov/health/educational/wecan/
news-events/matte1.htm.

13. Increased abdominal fat: Chronic: P. Björntorp, "Metabolic implications
of body fat distribution," *Diabetes Care* 14, no. 12 (Dec. 1991): 1132–43.
doi: 10.2337/diacare.14.12.1132. PMID: 1773700. https://pubmed.ncbi
.nlm.nih.gov/1773700/.

14. Research indicates that cortisol may influence: E. Epel, R. Lapidus,
B. McEwen, and K. Brownell, "Stress may add bite to appetite in women:
a laboratory study of stress-induced cortisol and eating behavior," *Psychoneuroendocrinology* 26, no. 1 (Jan. 2001): 37–49. doi: 10.1016/s0306
-4530(00)00035-4. PMID: 11070333. https://pubmed.ncbi.nlm.nih.gov/
11070333/.

15. Studies have shown that chronically: Jonathan Q. Purnell, Steven E. Kahn,
Mary H. Samuels, David Brandon, D. Lynn Loriaux, and John D. Brun-
zell, "Enhanced cortisol production rates, free cortisol, and 11ß-HSD-1
expression correlate with visceral fat and insulin resistance in men: effect
of weight loss," *American Journal of Physiology-Endocrinology and Metabolism* 296, no. 2 (Feb. 2009): E351–57. doi: 10.1152/ajpendo.90769.2008.
PMID: 19050176; PMCID: PMC2645022. https://www.ncbi.nlm.nih
.gov/pmc/articles/PMC2645022/.

16. Poor sleep quality and duration: Shahrad Taheri, Ling Lin, Diane Austin,
Terry Young, and Emmanuel Mignot, "Short sleep duration is associated
with reduced leptin, elevated ghrelin, and increased body mass index,"
PLoS Medicine 1, no. 3 (Dec. 2004): e62. doi: 10.1371/journal.pmed
.0010062. PMID: 15602591; PMCID: PMC535701. https://pubmed
.ncbi.nlm.nih.gov/15602591/.

17. Lower BMR may make it more: Ioannis Kyrou, George P. Chrousos,
and Constantine Tsigos, "Stress, visceral obesity, and metabolic complications," *Annals of the New York Academy of Sciences* 1083 (Nov. 2006):

77–110. doi: 10.1196/annals.1367.008. PMID: 17148735. https://pubmed.ncbi.nlm.nih.gov/17148735/.

18. Because repeated doses of caffeine: William R. Lovallo, Thomas L. Whitsett, Mustafa al'Absi, Bong Hee Sung, Andrea S. Vincent, and Michael F. Wilson, "Caffeine stimulation of cortisol secretion across the waking hours in relation to caffeine intake levels," *Psychosomatic Medicine* 67, no. 5 (Sept.–Oct. 2005): 734–39. doi: 10.1097/01.psy.0000181270.20036.06. PMID: 16204431; PMCID: PMC2257922. https://www.ncbi.nlm.nih.gov/pmc/articles/PMC2257922/.

19. Research published in *Environmental Research*: Gadi Lissak, "Adverse physiological and psychological effects of screen time on children and adolescents: literature review and case study," *Environmental Research* 164 (July 2018): 149–57. doi: 10.1016/j.envres.2018.01.015. PMID: 29499467. https://pubmed.ncbi.nlm.nih.gov/29499467/.

20. Breathing is one of the easiest: Howard E. LeWine, MD, "Relaxation techniques: Breath control helps quell errant stress response," Harvard Health Publishing/Harvard Medical School, July 24, 2024, https://www.health.harvard.edu/mind-and-mood/relaxation-techniques-breath-control-helps-quell-errant-stress-response.

21. Research suggests that even a single: Sebastian M. Schmid, Manfred Hallschmid, Kamila Jauch-Chara, Jan Born, and Bernd Schultes, "A single night of sleep deprivation increases ghrelin levels and feelings of hunger in normal-weight healthy men," *Journal of Sleep Research* 17, no. 3 (Sept. 2008): 331–34. doi: 10.1111/j.1365-2869.2008.00662.x. Epub 2008 Jun 28. PMID: 18564298. https://pubmed.ncbi.nlm.nih.gov/18564298/.

CHAPTER 9: GETTING PAST ROADBLOCKS AND DETOURS

1. Emotional eating: Positive moods can: Michael Macht, "How emotions affect eating: a five-way model," *Appetite* 50, no. 1 (Jan. 2008): 1–11. doi: 10.1016/j.appet.2007.07.002. PMID: 17707947. https://pubmed.ncbi.nlm.nih.gov/17707947/.

2. Hormonal influence: Mood fluctuations affect: E. Epel, R. Lapidus, B. McEwen, and K. Brownell, "Stress may add bite to appetite in women: a laboratory study of stress-induced cortisol and eating behavior," *Psychoneuroendocrinology* 26, no. 1 (Jan. 2001): 37–49. doi: 10.1016/s0306-4530(00)00035-4. PMID: 11070333. https://pubmed.ncbi.nlm.nih.gov/11070333/.

3. Preference shifts: Mood states alter: Alexander Fedorikhin and Vanessa M. Patrick, "Positive mood and resistance to temptation: the interfering influence of elevated arousal," *Journal of Consumer Research* 37, no. 4

(December 2010): 698–711. https://doi.org/10.1086/655665; https://academic.oup.com/jcr/article-abstract/37/4/698/1796848.

4. Metabolic effects: Stress-induced negative: Tanja C. Adam and Elissa S. Epel, "Stress, eating and the reward system," *Physiology & Behavior* 91, no. 4 (July 24, 2007): 449–58. https://www.sciencedirect.com/science/article/abs/pii/S0031938407001278.

5. Behavioral patterns: Chronic mood disturbances: Hanna Konttinen, Satu Männistö, Sirpo Sarlio-Lähteenkorva, Karri Silventoinen, and Ari Hauk-kala, "Emotional eating, depressive symptoms and self-reported food consumption. A population-based study," *Appetite* 54, no. 3 (June 2010): 473–79. doi: 10.1016/j.appet.2010.01.014. PMID: 20138944. https://pubmed.ncbi.nlm.nih.gov/20138944/.

6. Feeling depressed, meanwhile, can lead: Sarah E. Racine, Alexandra Burt, Pamela K. Keel, Cheryl L. Sisk, Michael C. Neale, Steven Boker et al., "Examining associations between negative urgency and key components of objective binge episodes," *International Journal of Eating Disorders*, April 10, 2015. https://doi.org/10.1002/eat.22412; https://onlinelibrary.wiley.com/doi/abs/10.1002/eat.22412.

7. When that stress becomes chronic: Harvard Health Publishing, Harvard Medical School, Staying Healthy, "Why stress causes people to overeat," February 15, 2021, https://www.health.harvard.edu/staying-healthy/why-stress-causes-people-to-overeat.

8. Your body will also secrete insulin: Mary F. Dallman, "Stress-induced obesity and the emotional nervous system," *Trends in Endocrinology & Metabolism* 21, no. 3 (Mar. 2010): 159–65. doi: 10.1016/j.tem.2009.10.004. PMID: 19926299; PMCID: PMC2831158. https://www.ncbi.nlm.nih.gov/pmc/articles/PMC2831158/.

9. Studies show that stress not only: Debra A. Zellner, Susan Loaiza, Zu-leyma Gonzalez, Jaclyn Pita, Janira Morales, Deanna Pecora et al., "Food selection changes under stress," *Physiology & Behavior* 87, no. 4 (Apr. 15, 2006): 789–93. doi: 10.1016/j.physbeh.2006.01.014. PMID: 16519909. https://pubmed.ncbi.nlm.nih.gov/16519909/.

10. Over time, persistent stress can: Matthew S. Tryon, Cameron S. Carter, Rashel Decant, and Kevin D. Laugero, "Chronic stress exposure may affect the brain's response to high calorie food cues and predispose to obesogenic eating habits," *Physiology & Behavior* 120 (Aug. 15, 2013): 233–42. doi: 10.1016/j.physbeh.2013.08.010. Epub 2013 Aug 16. PMID: 23954410. https://pubmed.ncbi.nlm.nih.gov/23954410/.

11. Your body tends to produce more: Karine Spiegel, Esra Tasali, Plamen Penev, and Eve Van Cauter, "Brief communication: sleep curtailment in healthy young men is associated with decreased leptin levels, elevated

ghrelin levels, and increased hunger and appetite," *Annals of Internal Medicine* 141, no. 11 (Dec. 7, 2004): 846–50. doi: 10.7326/0003-4819-141-11-200412070-00008. PMID: 15583226. https://pubmed.ncbi.nlm.nih.gov/15583226/.

12.   And studies have proven that you're: Yasmin Anwar, "Sleep deprivation linked to junk food cravings," UC Berkeley News, August 6, 2013, https://news.berkeley.edu/2013/08/06/poor-sleep-junk-food/.

13.   Although a single night of poor: Sebastian M. Schmid, Manfred Hallschmid, Kamila Jauch-Chara, Jan Born, and Bernd Schultes, "A single night of sleep deprivation increases ghrelin levels and feelings of hunger in normal-weight healthy men," *Journal of Sleep Research* 17, no. 3 (Sept. 2008): 331–34. doi: 10.1111/j.1365-2869.2008.00662.x. PMID: 18564298. https://pubmed.ncbi.nlm.nih.gov/18564298/.

14.   Numerous studies indicate that people: James E. Gangwisch, Dolores Malaspina, Bernadette Boden-Albala, and Steven B. Heymsfield, "Inadequate sleep as a risk factor for obesity: analyses of the NHANES I," *Sleep* 28, no. 10 (Oct. 2005): 1289–96. doi: 10.1093/sleep/28.10.1289. PMID: 16295214. https://pubmed.ncbi.nlm.nih.gov/16295214/.

15.   One study found that participants: Remco C. Havermans, Linda Vancleef, Antonis Kalamatianos, and Chantal Nederkoorn, "Eating and inflicting pain out of boredom," *Appetite* 85 (Feb. 2015): 52–57. doi: 10.1016/j.appet.2014.11.007. PMID: 25447018. https://pubmed.ncbi.nlm.nih.gov/25447018/.

16.   Another study found that people: Afton M. Koball, Molly R. Meers, Amy Storfer-Isser, Sarah E. Domoff, and Dara R. Musher-Eizenman, "Eating when bored: revision of the emotional eating scale with a focus on boredom," *Health Psychology* 31, no. 4 (July 2012): 521–24. doi: 10.1037/a0025893. PMID: 22004466. https://pubmed.ncbi.nlm.nih.gov/22004466/.

17.   One meta-analysis of twenty-four studies: Eric Robinson, Paul Aveyard, Amanda Daley, Kate Jolly, Amanda Lewis, Deborah Lycett et al., "Eating attentively: a systematic review and meta-analysis of the effect of food intake memory and awareness on eating," *American Journal of Clinical Nutrition* 97, no. 4 (Apr. 2013): 728–42. doi: 10.3945/ajcn.112.045245. PMID: 23446890; PMCID: PMC3607652. https://pubmed.ncbi.nlm.nih.gov/23446890/.

18.   Conversely, a different study found that women: Eric Robinson, Inge Kersbergen, and Suzanne Higgs, "Eating 'attentively' reduces later energy consumption in overweight and obese females," *British Journal of Nutrition* 112, no. 4 (Aug. 28, 2014): 657–61. doi: 10.1017/S000711451400141X. PMID: 24933322. https://pubmed.ncbi.nlm.nih.gov/24933322/.

19. Researchers have found that your: L. A. De Luca, Jr., R. C. Vendramini, D. T. Pereira, D. A. Colombari, R. B. David, P. M. de Paula et al., "Water deprivation and the double-depletion hypothesis: common neural mechanisms underlie thirst and salt appetite," *Brazilian Journal of Medical and Biological Research* 40, no. 5 (May 2007): 707–12. doi: 10.1590/s0100-879x2007000500015. PMID: 17464434. https://pubmed.ncbi.nlm.nih.gov/17464434/.

20. You might not be aware of your "neural mechanisms": Carolina Dalmasso, José Antunes-Rodrigues, Laura Vivas, and Laurival A. De Luca, Jr., "Mapping brain Fos immunoreactivity in response to water deprivation and partial rehydration: influence of sodium intake," *Physiology & Behavior* 151 (Nov. 1, 2015): 494–501. doi: 10.1016/j.physbeh.2015.08.020. PMID: 26297688. https://pubmed.ncbi.nlm.nih.gov/26297688/.

21. Follow Harvard's *The Nutrition Source*: Harvard T. H. Chan School of Public Health, The Nutrition Source, "3 strategies to prevent overeating," January 13, 2015, https://nutritionsource.hsph.harvard.edu/2015/01/13/3-strategies-to-prevent-overeating/.

22. Also, chew more—increased: Eric Robinson, Eva Almiron-Roig, Femke Rutters, Cees de Graaf, Ciarán G. Forde, Catrin Tudur Smith et al., "A systematic review and meta-analysis examining the effect of eating rate on energy intake and hunger," *American Journal of Clinical Nutrition* 100, no. 1 (July 2014): 123–51. doi: 10.3945/ajcn.113.081745. PMID: 24847856. https://pubmed.ncbi.nlm.nih.gov/24847856/.

CHAPTER 10: KICK-START TWO-WEEK MEAL PLAN

1. In fact, vegetarians may need. Rose Carr, "Why do vegetarians need more protein?" Healthy Food Guide, April 3, 2017, https://www.healthyfood.com/advice/why-do-vegetarians-need-more-protein/.

Index

About the Author

Harley Pasternak is an adjunct professor at the University of Toronto and holds a master of science in exercise physiology and nutritional sciences from the same university. He also holds an honors degree in kinesiology from the University of Western Ontario and served as an exercise and nutrition scientist for Canada's Department of National Defence.

Pasternak is a *New York Times* bestselling author whose books include *5-Factor Fitness*, *The 5-Factor Diet*, *The 5-Factor World Diet*, *The Body Reset Diet*, *The Body Reset Diet Cookbook*, and *5 Pounds*. Harley's titles have attained global bestseller status, which has resulted in translations into fourteen languages in more than twenty-five countries around the world.

As a fitness and nutrition specialist, Pasternak boasts the largest celebrity client roster in the industry, and has worked with Ariana Grande, Lady Gaga, Rihanna, Halle Berry, Katy Perry, Megan Fox, Robert Downey, Jr., Robert Pattinson, Jessica Simpson, Gwen Stefani, Adam Levine, Kim Kardashian, John Mayer, Alicia Keys, and Jennifer Hudson.

Harley starred on *Revenge Body with Khloé Kardashian* on E! and was a regular contributor to *Good Morning America* on ABC. Harley has also been featured as a judge on *America's Next Top Model*, hosted *The Revolution* on ABC, and starred as himself in the 2014 feature film *Teenage Mutant Ninja Turtles*.

Pasternak has made worldwide speaking appearances in more than thirty countries for a range of Fortune 500 companies, health and fitness organizations, and government entities. He is a Toronto native and currently resides with his wife and two children in Los Angeles.

01 14